A Guide to

# The Practice of Nursing using the Nursing Process

Dedicated to the staff and students in the Department of Nursing, University of Manchester, and to the patients and staff of the Manchester Royal Infirmary

# A Guide to
# The Practice of Nursing
# using the Nursing Process

## Baroness McFarlane of Llandaff

Hon D Sc (Ulster), MA (Lond.), Hon M Sc (Manch.), B Sc (Soc.) (Lond.),
SRN, SCM, HV Tut Cert FRCN

Professor and Head of Department of Nursing,
University of Manchester

## George Castledine

M Sc (Manch.), BA, Dip Soc Sc (Oxon), SRN, FRCN

Clinical Lecturer,
Manchester Royal Infirmary and Department of
Nursing, University of Manchester

# The C.V. Mosby Company

London · St Louis · Toronto 1982

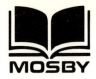

**MOSBY**

A TRADITION OF PUBLISHING EXCELLENCE

C.V. Mosby Publication
Mosby – Yearbook Ltd,
Barnard's Inn, Holborn, London EC1N 2JA

**British Library Cataloguing in Publication Data**

McFarlane of Llandaff, Jean Kennedy McFarlane,
*Baroness*
A guide to the practice of nursing using the
nursing process.
1. Nursing
I. Title        II. Castledine, George
610.73    RT41

ISBN 0-8016-3278-1

**Library of Congress Cataloguing in Publication Data**

McFarlane of Llandaff, Jean Kennedy McFarlane,
   Baroness, 1926–
A guide to the practice of nursing using the
nursing process.

Bibliography: p.
Includes index.
   1. Nursing.   I. Castledine, George.   II. Title
|DNLM: 1. Nursing process.   2. Patient care
planning. WY 100 M478g]
RT41.M474          610.73        82-7837
ISBN 0-8016-3278-1                    AACR2

Printed in Great Britain by
St Edmundsbury Press Ltd, Bury St Edmunds, Suffolk
Bound by Dorstel Press, Harlow and London

# Preface

In 1973, the Department of Nursing in the University of Manchester held a staff seminar on the 'nursing process'. Since then, the use of this systematic approach to the planning of nursing care has become an important element in its educational and clinical work. Planning nursing care by use of the nursing process was first introduced in the course leading to the Diploma in Advanced Nursing Studies for experienced registered nurses. It was then gradually introduced into the undergraduate (Bachelor of Nursing) programme. Increasing familiarity with the process has led to its use as a basis for identifying curriculum content and in assessing the clinical competence of students. These educational uses would be little more than academic exercises unless the department had found a clinical setting in which it could test the validity of the approach in practice. This it has been able to do, by creating joint appointments between the department and the National Health Service. In 1976, two members of staff were appointed as clinical lecturers, that is they worked half time as a ward sister or charge nurse at Manchester Royal Infirmary and half time as lecturers in the Department of Nursing. Thus, between them they carried out the work of one lecturer and one ward sister. The first appointments were in an acute traumatic surgery unit.

After three years the posts were transferred to a newly opened geriatric assessment unit. A further joint appointment has recently been established in midwifery. In these first joint appointments it has been possible to develop and test the use of the nursing process.

The department is often asked for an account of the work it has done in this respect. Articles by Ashworth, Castledine and McFarlane (1978) and Ashworth and Castledine (1980) have described it. This book is an attempt to describe the approach used in greater detail. It is written at a simple level and is intended for students entering the nursing profession, or for trained nurses who have not previously used the nursing process. The more one uses the 'process', however, the more profound its implications become for clinical practice, the management of patient care, education and research.

In Part I we outline the system of values and beliefs we have about the nature of the nursing function, since it is these which determine the content of nursing care plans; the stages in the nursing process are then outlined. In Part II a description is given of the way in which the process has been used in the clinical unit associated with the Department of Nursing in the University of Manchester.

We would like to acknowledge the University of Manchester, Department of Medical Illustration, for the excellent photographs used in the book.

# Authors' Note

For the sake of verisimilitude we have included names of doctors, nursing staff, patients and patients' relatives and friends on several of the charts and care notes. These are entirely fictitious names and do not refer to actual people, living or dead.

# Contents

# Part I

## NURSING AND THE NURSING PROCESS IN PRINCIPLE

## Introduction

The practice of nursing is shaped by the values and ideas which nurses and others hold of their own function. Nursing is such a complex activity that it is virtually impossible to find a simple definition for so wide a range of actions. It is necessary, however, if nursing actions are to be integrated and goal-directed, to give some thought to its nature and characteristics; what it is and what it is not. This is done by setting out a series of statements about nursing and giving an analysis of the elements which are in any nursing situation. At the end of Part I, the process of planning nursing care is outlined and then, in Part II, the practicalities of care planning are dealt with.

**1**

# The Nature and Characteristics
# of Nursing

Before setting out to make a systematic plan of nursing care for an individual (or community) there is a need to clarify what is meant by nursing, that is, what one is planning. The word 'nursing' has different derivations and meanings in different languages, and in some languages there is no word for it. Although there may be a common core of function, in different cultures the role and functions of the nurse vary widely. As the Report of the Committee on Nursing (DHSS, 1972) indicated, there are public and professional images of the work of the nurse which are sometimes at variance with the reality of nursing as it is practised.

   In our own society, nursing is part of a health-care system within a welfare state; it is a complex human activity which defies a simple definition. It is perhaps best described by a series of statements about its properties which contribute to our understanding of its nature:

1. Nursing and health care in our society owe much to their historical antecedents — to Christian and philanthropic foundations and provisions through the Poor Law and local government. The present health-care system is part of a complex of inter-related provisions by the state which includes social security and education. Provisions are made through insurance and taxation, and the initial vision of the National Health Service (which has been eroded with the passage of time) was that services should be free at the time of use.
   *Nursing is culturally and economically determined.*

2. Within a complex health service, having functions ranging from organ transplant to farm management in hospitals for the mentally handi-capped, there is a great range of specialisation in roles. Within this system nursing has a far more specialised role than it may have, for instance, in a Third World country, where such differentiation of health-care roles would be inappropriate. In our society the nursing and medical roles are differentiated but there is a degree of overlap.
   *In a complex society, nursing is differentiated and specialised as a health-care role.*

3. By derivation, the word to 'nurse' means to 'nourish', as when a mother feeds a baby. Some fundamental insights into the nature of nursing are given in this origin which demonstrates its distinction from the medical role.
   *The root meaning of the word to 'nurse' is to 'nourish'.*

4. By extension, nursing has to do with meeting other basic human needs for life and health such as fluids, shelter, sleep and rest, love, belonging, etc. These can be categorised as physiological, psychological, and social needs.
   *Nursing has to do with meeting basic human needs for life and health.*

5. These basic human needs are normally met by the individual carrying out 'activities of daily living' or 'self-care' (Henderson, 1966; Orem, 1980).
   *Basic human needs are normally met by the activities of daily living or self-care.*

6. The infant being fed by its mother is by reason of age unable to get nourishment for himself, i.e. there is a deficiency in the ability of the baby to meet its own nutritional needs as an adult could. Nursing has to do with meeting deficiencies in the abilities of people to meet their own basic physiological or psychosocial needs. There are deficits in the ability to carry out self-care.
   *Nursing has to do with meeting the deficiencies of people in carrying out daily living activities, i.e. with deficits in self-care ability.*

7. A baby cannot meet his own nutritional needs by reason of age — he is not developmentally ready for the task of foraging for food or buying in the market place. Similarly, elderly people may lose the ability to meet their own basic needs. Disease or its treatment may also affect the ability of individuals to meet their own needs, as may ignorance or lack of motivation.
   *The deficiencies in ability to meet one's own basic needs with which nursing deals may be caused by developmental immaturity, deterioration in function, disease, disability, diagnostic and therapeutic regimes, ignorance or poor motivation.*

8. The lack of ability in self-care varies in degree. It may be such as to produce total dependence on another, or others, for care. It may demand a minor degree of physical or psychological or social support, or be aided by counselling, teaching or change of environment. One of the skills of nursing is to assess the extent of deficiency in ability for self-care, the extent to which the individual, the family or society may be

able to make good the deficiency, and the extent to which skilled nursing intervention is needed.
*Deficiencies in self-care vary in kind and degree which have to be assessed.*

9.  In the mother meeting the nutritional needs of a baby is a picture of mutuality and reciprocity in which the mother assesses needs, provides a secure environment and gives nourishment, while the child indicates need and works in sucking to meet that need. Later in life, as the child is weaned, different criteria for assessment and provision are used and the child develops increasing sophistication and independence in meeting his own need. Nursing takes over, helps or promotes the self-caring activities for another person or a community. The degree of need has constantly to be reassessed and the respective roles of nurse and patient will develop and change as the patient regains ability to maintain a sufficient quantity and quality of self-care. There is always a reciprocal relationship involved and the patient has a right to contribute to the decision-making about his care.
    *Nursing is essentially a reciprocal and dynamically changing re-lationship between patient and nurse. The activities of nursing give help or assistance with a view to promoting and maximising the self-care abilities of the individual or community.*

10. Deficits in ability to meet the basic needs for life and health may be actual or potential. There is a well-defined nursing role in promoting the quality and quantity of self-care requisite for health. This includes not only imparting knowledge about ways of meeting the basic human needs for life and health, but also motivating individuals and societies to utilise that knowledge in health-promoting and disease-preventing activities, i.e. in education for health.
    *There is a nursing role in educating for health, i.e. aiding in health promotion and disease prevention.*

11. Nursing is not just an activity directed at the health and well-being of individuals. The health of communities is as vital and the two are intimately related. Nursing is concerned with health promotion, disease prevention and assistance in self-care activities of communities.
    *Nursing has to do with the self-caring activities of both individuals and communities and their inter-relationship.*

12. Those factors which may precipitate the need for nursing intervention (deficiencies in self-caring ability caused by developmental immaturity, deterioration of function, disease or therapy, ignorance or lack of motivation) may cause a permanent or progressive state of impairment in the ability to meet basic human needs. Restoration to full self-care

may not be a realistic goal. Even when nursing intervention is consistently required to maintain the daily living activities, it is possible to maximise the contribution of the individual in self-care. In long-term care and in the process of dying it is important that the dignity of the individual should be preserved as far as possible by helping him to maximise his self-care ability and, in the end, to help him to die in a way which expresses his personality and beliefs.

*In some situations where it is not possible to regain full ability in self-care, nursing maintains the self-care function and maximises the contribution of the individual, helping him in the end to die with dignity and expressing his personality.*

# SUMMARY OF STATEMENTS ABOUT THE NATURE OF NURSING

1. Nursing is culturally and economically determined.

2. In a complex society, nursing is differentiated and specialised as a health-care role.

3. The root meaning of the word to 'nurse' is to 'nourish'.

4. Nursing has to do with meeting basic human needs for life and health.

5. Basic human needs are normally met by activities of daily living or self-care.

6. Nursing has to do with meeting the deficiencies of people in carrying out daily living activities, i.e. with deficits in self-care ability.

7. The deficiencies in ability to meet one's own basic needs with which nursing deals may be caused by developmental immaturity, deterioration in function, disease, disability, diagnostic and therapeutic regimes, ignorance or poor motivation.

8. Deficiencies in self-care vary in kind and degree which have to be assessed.

9. Nursing is essentially a reciprocal and dynamically changing relationship between patient and nurse. The activities of nursing give help or assistance with a view to promoting and maximising the self-care abilities of the individual or community.

10. There is a nursing role in educating for health, i.e. aiding in health promotion and disease prevention.

11. Nursing has to do with the self-caring activities of both individuals and communities and their inter-relationship.

12. In some situations where it is not possible to regain full ability in self-care, nursing maintains the self-care function and maximises the contribution of the individual, helping him in the end to die with dignity and expressing his personality.

# The Elements of Nursing — A Conceptual Framework

In the 12 statements made about nursing in Chapter 1, four inter-related elements occur which can be brought together into a conceptual framework:

1. Man.
2. Society.
3. Health.
4. Nursing.

These elements can be represented diagrammatically, as shown in *Figure 2.1*, and described as follows:

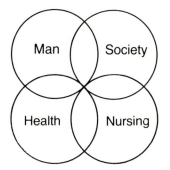

**Figure 2.1**   Conceptual framework for nursing

1. *Man.* The individual person has physiological, psychological and social aspects to his make-up; that is, he is a physio-psychosocial being. He has basic needs for the preservation of life and health. Maslow (1954) has presented these as a hierarchy; that is, one class of need must be satisfied before subsequent levels can be met:

(a) Physiological or survival needs.
(b) Security and safety needs.
(c) Belonging or affection needs.
(d) Self-esteem or respect needs.
(e) Self-actualisation.

**Society**

2. *Society*. Physical provisions such as housing and environmental health services (sewage and refuse disposal, etc.) are an essential element in health provision and intimately affect the health of individuals, but sociological factors also determine the way in which health and illness are defined in a society and the way in which its health services are organised and made available. In our society there is a class differential in the way in which health services are utilised (Black, 1980). The organisation of the nursing service is culturally determined and derives much from its historical roots in maternal, religious and military roles, and the position of women in society (Davies, 1980).

**Health**

3. *Health*. Nursing operates in the health field. The definition of health by the World Health Organisation (1947) as 'not merely the absence of disease but a state of complete mental, physical and social well-being' is now regarded as being somewhat idealistic. In the USA, the President's Commission on the Health Needs of the Nation (1953) gave a more realistic and dynamic view of health: '. . . it is not a condition, it is an adjustment. It is not a state, but a process. The process adapts the individual not only to our physical but also our social environment.' Dunn (1961) drew attention to the fact that different individuals have different levels of wellness. The optimum for the individual he called 'high level wellness', which he defined as an 'integrated method of functioning which is oriented toward maximising the

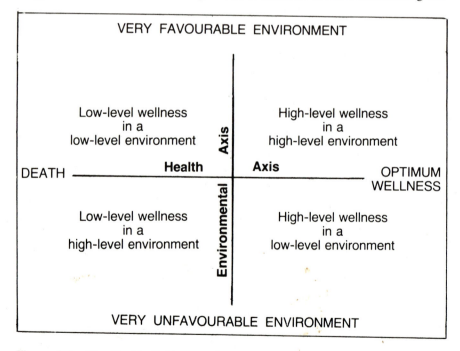

**Figure 2.2**   The Health Grid (from Dunn, 1958)

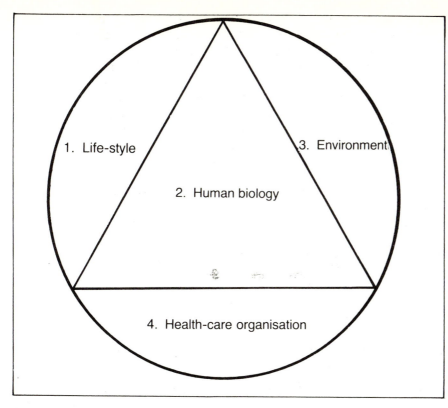

*Figure 2.3*   The Health Field concept (after Lalonde, 1974)

potential of which the individual is capable, within the environment where he is functioning'. He describes two axes of well-being: a health axis (from death to optimum wellness) and an environmental axis (from very unfavourable to favourable). His Health Grid (*Figure 2.2*) shows levels of wellness in relation to health and environment (Dunn, 1958).

The Canadian Minister of National Health and Welfare (Lalonde, 1974), put forward the Health Field concept (*Figure 2.3*) which identified four broad elements underlying the health of the population; these are, life-style, human biology, environment and health-care organisation. Lalonde (1974) suggested that 'protecting the food supply from contamination, and drugs from being abused, as well as recognising alcohol abuse, smoking, obesity, lack of physical fitness, chronic illness, venereal disease, and traffic deaths are national health problems', and open to government initiatives.

4. *Nursing*. This is a complex human activity which assists the individual or a society in the promotion and maintenance of those activities which contribute to health and well-being, with particular reference to basic human physiological, psychological and social needs. These needs are normally met

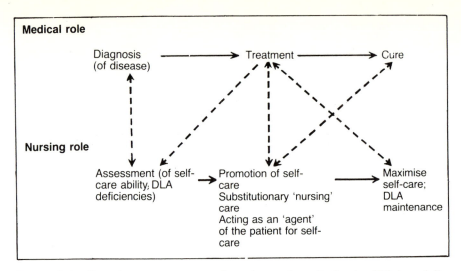

***Figure 2.4***   Complementary nature of nursing and medical roles (DLA = daily
living activities)

by daily living activities carried out by the individual (self-care), but much
nursing care of an unskilled type is carried out by families and friends. Where
deficiencies in self-care are of such a nature or of such an order that the
individual, or the family, is unable to maintain a sufficient quantity or quality
of self-care, then skilled and professional nursing intervention is required.
The practice of professional nursing is in a colleague relationship with that of
the practice of medicine and other health professions. Promoting and
maintaining daily living activities forms a back-cloth to all other health
activities. They maintain the human organism while other health professionals intervene to diagnose and treat disease. Nursing provides the
environment for the maintenance of life which makes all other health
functions possible. In a complex health system, nursing has this essential and
distinctive role to play alongside that of other health workers. The nurse is
the authority on the maintenance of daily living activities while the doctor is,
for instance, the authority on the diagnosis and treatment of disease. The
roles are complementary and so closely related as to prohibit an adversarial
relationship. *Figure 2.4* is a diagrammatic representation of the close
relationship of the medical and nursing roles.

Although the distinctive features of each role are shown in the diagram,
there is clearly a great deal of reference between the doctor and nurse in
planning patient care, and there is often overlap and interchangeability of
roles. The nurse often assists in diagnostic tests and therapeutic regimes, but
her major function is in maintaining the daily living activities and environmental needs contributing to health and well-being. For the chronic sick or
the elderly these needs may be all the health care they require. For others,
they form the back-cloth against which medical intervention can take place.

**3**

# The Process of Planning Nursing Care — the Nursing Process

## Elements of a nursing care planning system

Having analysed the elements involved in nursing it is necessary to develop a systematic method for making decisions about what nursing care is needed and planning how it should be carried out. The system needs to provide a way of identifying:

1. The individual deficits in self-care and their causes, i.e. the patient's problems.

2. The objectives or expected outcomes of nursing care.

3. Nursing methods for promoting or maintaining self-care activities or substituting for deficiencies in self-care.

4. Plans for implementing the methods.

5. The effectiveness of the care given.

In much of the literature, this systematic approach to decision-making and planning nursing care is called 'the nursing process'. Some writers prefer to talk about 'a systematic approach to planning nursing care'. There is a common recognition that certain stages must be passed through in planning nursing care.

### *Advantages of using the nursing process*

The current emphasis on systematic planning is an attempt to improve the quality of that planning, to place the decision-making on a more scientific basis, and to evaluate the outcomes more effectively. By contrast with previous approaches to planning, use of the nursing process attempts to:

1. Assess patient needs on an individualised rather than routinised basis.

2. Provide a basis for analysis of the causes of patient needs so that the nursing actions planned can be related more closely to the problems.

3. Provide a system for analysing the individual's or the family's ability to sustain self-care and to review the professional intervention needed.

4. Document or write down the plan and record of treatment as a means of staff communication.

5. Make explicit the nursing actions planned to meet particular patient problems so that their effectiveness can be reviewed.

6. Provide a method of evaluating nursing care.

# Stages in the nursing process

Although different nurses identify varying numbers of stages in the nursing process and give the stages different names, most of them are in effect describing the same thing. The differences depend on how finely the steps or stages in planning are divided. For the purposes of this book, the *five* stages outlined are those used in the original Manchester staff seminar paper:

1. Data collection.

2. Assessment.

3. Planning.

4. Implementation.

5. Evaluation.

(Nurses working with the World Health Organisation medium term programme on the nursing process will recognise that 'data collection' is incorporated in the 'assessment' stage, and *four* stages are used.)

These five stages are inter-related (*Figure 3.1*) and there is need for reassessment and modification of plans as evaluation takes place. The process is best regarded, therefore, as circular (*Figure 3.2*).

In this chapter an overview is given of each stage in the nursing process. In Part II (Chapters 4–9) the practical implications of the five stages are examined in greater depth.

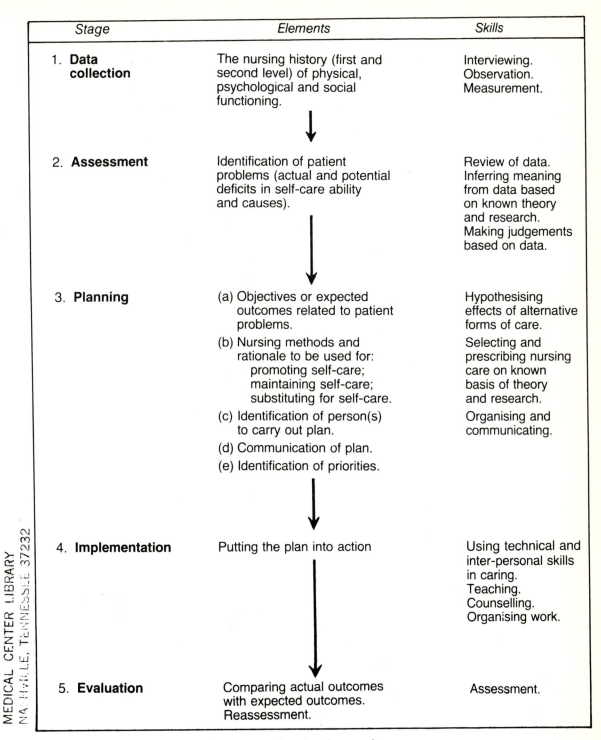

| Stage | Elements | Skills |
|-------|----------|--------|
| 1. **Data collection** | The nursing history (first and second level) of physical, psychological and social functioning. | Interviewing. Observation. Measurement. |
| 2. **Assessment** | Identification of patient problems (actual and potential deficits in self-care ability and causes). | Review of data. Inferring meaning from data based on known theory and research. Making judgements based on data. |
| 3. **Planning** | (a) Objectives or expected outcomes related to patient problems.<br>(b) Nursing methods and rationale to be used for: promoting self-care; maintaining self-care; substituting for self-care.<br>(c) Identification of person(s) to carry out plan.<br>(d) Communication of plan.<br>(e) Identification of priorities. | Hypothesising effects of alternative forms of care.<br>Selecting and prescribing nursing care on known basis of theory and research.<br>Organising and communicating. |
| 4. **Implementation** | Putting the plan into action | Using technical and inter-personal skills in caring. Teaching. Counselling. Organising work. |
| 5. **Evaluation** | Comparing actual outcomes with expected outcomes. Reassessment. | Assessment. |

**Figure 3.1**   Essential elements in a system for planning nursing care

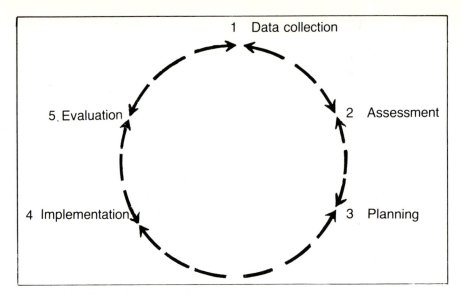

*Figure 3.2*   Stages in the nursing process

## Stage 1: Data collection

| *Elements* | *Skills* |
|---|---|
| The nursing history (first and second level) of physical, pyschological and social functioning. | Interviewing. Observation. Measurement. |

To plan nursing care effectively the nurse needs to be able to assess the individual's needs for nursing care; that is, to identify where there are problems of maintaining a sufficient quantity and quality of self-care activity for health and well-being. To make this assessment, information is needed on all aspects of functioning. Taking a holistic or total person approach to nursing care implies that information is needed about physiological, psychological and social functioning.

Information could be gathered on the basis of presenting, or obvious, problems. There are deficiencies in this approach; the patient may not volunteer or the nurse may not observe a fundamental problem unless a systematic screening of self-care abilities takes place. The psychological and social problems would inevitably be neglected by comparison with more obvious physical problems. The first stage in planning, therefore, is systematic information gathering or collecting data about the patient's self-care abilities. A nursing history is a tool for this systematic data collection. It may be set out as a series of questions on different aspects of functional ability.

Some nursing history formats contain pre-set questions which either demand a tick in a box or a simple answer. For example:

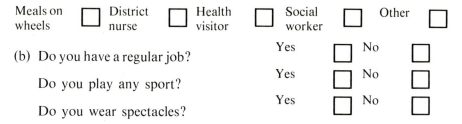

(a) Have you been receiving any of the following services at home?

Meals on
wheels ☐    District
nurse ☐    Health
visitor ☐    Social
worker ☐    Other ☐

(b) Do you have a regular job?            Yes ☐    No ☐

    Do you play any sport?                Yes ☐    No ☐

    Do you wear spectacles?               Yes ☐    No ☐

Some people feel that a list of questions is too restrictive and prefer to have headings so that the information about, for example, the function of elimination, can be gained by free and conversational methods. Whatever the approach, a checklist of items to be covered needs to be developed and the nursing history form should be designed so that a record can be made as a means of communication to other nurses.

The content of the nursing history will deal with daily living activities such as eating, sleeping, breathing, eliminating, etc.

Some nurses use the following 14 activities as a checklist for data collection (Henderson, 1966):

1. Breathe normally.

2. Eat and drink adequately.

3. Eliminate body wastes.

4. Move and maintain desirable postures.

5. Sleep and rest.

6. Select suitable clothes — dress and undress.

7. Maintain body temperature within normal range by adjusting clothing and modifying the environment.

8. Keep the body clean and well groomed and protect the integument.

9. Avoid danger in the environment and avoid injuring others.

10. Communicate with others in expressing emotions, needs, fear or opinions.

11. Worship according to one's faith.

12. Work in such a way that there is a sense of accomplishment.

13. Play or participate in various forms of recreation.

14. Learn, discover or satisfy the curiosity that leads to normal development and health and use the available health facilities.

McCain (1965) lists 13 areas for data collection, of which the following four are examples:

*Mental status*
    State of consciousness
    Orientation
    Intellectual capacity
    Attention span
    Vocabulary level
    Ability to understand ideas

*Emotional status*
    Emotional reactions
    Body image
    Ability to relate to others

*Sensory perception*
    Hearing
    Vision
    Speech
    Touch
    Smell
    Taste

*Motor ability*
    Mobility
    Range of motion
    Gait
    Equilibrium
    Muscle tone
    Paralysis
    Loss of extremity

For each heading, McCain spells out descriptive statements which are aids to identifying the status of the patient in given abilities; for example:

*State of consciousness*
    Alert and quick to respond to surroundings
    Drowsy and slow to respond
    Semiconscious and difficult to arouse
    Comatose and unable to arouse
    State of automatism

In Part II we describe how the nursing history is taken in two stages in the geriatric assessment ward at Manchester Royal Infirmary. Headings such as 'Activity', 'Rest', 'Nutrition', etc., are given and information is gathered in unstructured interviews. To help nurses in the early stages of its use, a teaching aid with prompts about the content to be covered is given (see *Figure 4.4*).

It is likely that the student of nursing will find that the format of the nursing history has been developed on the wards where she works. It does no harm to try to develop a format of one's own, to use different approaches, and to try to improve on those that have been developed. The nursing care plan will probably be as effective as the assessment made, and a great deal depends on how good the nursing history is.

## Normal functioning and ability to cope with dysfunction

The patient's ability to carry out the daily living activities associated with health are reviewed to get information about:

1. How the patient normally carries out each function. The nursing care plan should aim to assist the patient to carry out these activities as nearly as possible to the way in which he normally carries them out, so that self-care can be maintained or re-established as quickly as possible.
2. The nature and extent of deviation from normal functioning for the individual at that time. This will vary from time to time and hence there is need to reassess the functional ability at intervals.
3. The ability of the individual to adapt to limited dysfunction and maintain self-care; for example, the ability of the patient with arthritis to dress himself using artificial aids, or the ability of the patient with pre-operative anxiety to express it.

The second stage nursing history form illustrated in Chapter 4 (see *Figure 4.7*) allows the nurse to record the 'Usual condition/behaviour' and the 'Present condition/behaviour'. By comparing and contrasting what is normal for that individual with the present behaviour, the nurse is able to form a judgement about whether any aspect of daily living activity presents a problem to the patient. This is the first stage in making an assessment. For example:

| Usual condition/behaviour (or normal self-care behaviour) | Present condition/behaviour (or disabilities in self-care) |
|---|---|
| Able to dress himself. | Unable to make fine adjustments in clothing (do/undo back zips fully, tie shoelaces, etc). |
| Able to maintain personal hygiene. | Unable to wash 'good' arm because of immobilisation of one arm in plaster. |

Besides the detailed information about daily living activities, more general background information is needed about the patient. Information such as his name and how he prefers to be addressed, what he understands about his condition and his reaction to hospital admission are basic to any further communication.

### The skills of data collection

Taking a nursing history is one of the most skilled nursing functions. Information about the patient is gathered by observation and communication. Observation includes a superficial assessment of the patient's colour, skin condition, muscle tone, etc., and recorded observations such as temperature, pulse, respirations and blood pressure, and may include a more detailed physical examination. Communications may be with the patient himself, his family or friends, and with other health professionals. They may be written or spoken (see *Figures 5.1, 5.2 and 5.3*).

The skill of communicating with a patient is fundamental to nursing practice and is more complex than many manual skills. It includes controlling the environment so that effective communication can take place, the art of listening and the ability to allow the patient to express anxieties and fears and intimate facts. Whenever personal details are being sought or emotional problems come to light, there is a professional and ethical need to preserve the confidentiality of the information and to avoid probing into private affairs out of mere curiosity. The information needed is that on which an adequate plan of nursing care can be built.

## Stage 2: Assessment

| Elements | Skills |
|---|---|
| Identification of patient problems (actual and potential deficits in self-care ability and causes). | Review of data. Inferring meaning from data based on known theory and research. Making judgements based on data. |

As indicated above, the object of gathering information is the identification of patient problems with daily living activities.

The nursing history is not an end in itself — it is a tool to elicit and record information so that problems can be identified and plans made to deal with them. Taking a nursing history is, then, only the first stage in the nursing process and of little value in its own right. Having collected the information, the intellectual skill of assessment takes place. Involved in this are:

(a) Review of the information.
(b) Making of inferences about its significance.
(c) Identification of problems.

A nursing history yields a great deal of information. In order to use it as a basis for care planning there is need to review it, comparing it with normal functioning. To do this, a knowledge of normal anatomical, physiological, psychological and social functioning is needed. A comparison of normal functioning is made with the information gathered about normal functioning for that individual and the present abilities in daily living activities. From this review of scientific knowledge and the individual's experience, certain inferences may be drawn. We may infer that the individual can cope with some deviations from normal functioning himself, but other self-care activities may not be maintained at an optimum level. These are identified as 'patient problems', for which a plan of nursing care must be designed. The end of the assessment stage, therefore, is the identification of patient problems and these become the basis of the care plan. Both actual and potential problems (not present, but which may occur) will feature in the list.

For example, in reviewing a case of normal self-care behaviour in dressing and personal hygiene, with the observed behaviour and reported disabilities, certain patient problems are identified:

(a) Problem with fine adjustments in dressing.
(b) Problem with washing 'good' arm due to immobilisation of arm.

Here there are actual problems for which a plan of care must be devised.

A further example could concern an elderly person at home who may have difficulty in preparing meals because of a loss of motivation or mobility. She has a potential problem of malnutrition which needs to be incorporated in her plan of care.

Note that the problems identified are those of the patient, not the nurse!

## Stage 3: Planning

| Elements | Skills |
|---|---|
| (a) Objectives or expected outcomes related to patient problems. | Hypothesising effects of alternative forms of care. |
| (b) Nursing methods and rationale to be used for: promoting self-care; maintaining self-care; substituting for self-care. | Selecting and prescribing nursing care on known basis of theory and research. |
| (c) Identification of person(s) to carry out plan. | Organising |
| (d) Communication of plan. | and |
| (e) Identification of priorities. | communicating |

A systematic plan of care for an individual patient should have the following elements:

1. A statement of actual and potential problems.

2. The objectives or expected outcomes of nursing care for each problem.

3. Prescription of nursing actions to achieve the objectives.

## 1. *Statement of problems*

At the end of the assessment stage a list of patient problems with daily living activities should have been identified. There will be actual problems presented at the time of taking the nursing history, but also potential problems will be identified; that is, those which may occur if preventive action is not taken. The problems need to be listed in some order of priority for action (life-saving actions would obviously be urgent), but it is also worth while to indicate very briefly what the cause of the problem is. For example, 'potential problem of pressure sores due to inability to move freely in bed'. The cause of the problem gives some indication as to the kind of nursing action required to overcome it.

## 2. *Objectives or expected outcomes*

The next stage in planning is to state briefly what kind of patient outcome the nurse and patient together decide they wish to achieve for each problem. Just as problems are identified by observing or communicating with the patient, so after nursing care has been carried out one should be able to observe or find out from the patient what the effects or outcomes of the care have been. For example, for a patient with a problem of dehydration due to insufficient fluid intake by mouth, one might set an objective or expected outcome of $2\frac{1}{2}$ litres of fluid intake in 24 hours. One can then observe whether that outcome is achieved.

One may also observe the non-verbal cues of facial expression, colour and reduction in restlessness which may be the expected outcomes in nursing care designed to relieve anxiety. The patient himself may report on the outcomes of nursing care designed to relieve sleeplessness or constipation.

The expected outcomes, therefore, are stated in terms of patient behaviour rather than nursing action. They form an important basis for evaluating nursing care, so the more precisely they are stated, the more effective they will be. It is useful, whenever possible, to quantify the expected outcomes and the period of time for their achievement (deadlines) — the example given above, '$2\frac{1}{2}$ litres in 24 hours', illustrates this. It is important that as far as possible the patient is involved in the decisions about his care.

## 3. *Nursing actions*

The third element in the care plan is a concise statement of the nursing actions designed to achieve the desired outcomes of nursing care, how these should be carried out and how frequently. For example, for the patient with a potential problem of pressure sores due to inability to move freely in bed, expected outcomes might be set:

'No skin breakdown at buttocks or elbows.'

and the prescribed nursing action might be:

'Turn 2 hourly (10 a.m., 12 midday, 2 p.m., 4 p.m., 6 p.m., 8 p.m., etc.).'

For a patient with a problem of grief due to death of a spouse, objectives might be:

'Ability to talk about loss, to express emotions, to regain involvement in personal affairs.'

The nursing actions might include:

'Allow patient to express emotions, allow privacy and time to be alone, be positive about regaining personal involvement.'

Prescribing nursing actions which will provide an effective solution to patient problems is the heart of professional nursing practice. Manual dexterity in nursing is important of course, but unless nursing actions are effectively aimed at the individual patient problem and have a sound rationale they may be dangerous or, at best, a waste of time.

The prescription of nursing actions can only be effective if the nurse has a knowledge of the physiological, psychological and social basis of the deficits in self-care that the patient is experiencing. A knowledge of the effects of disease on some daily living activities may require a knowledge of pathophysiology. The nurse, then, needs to be able to review possible alternative forms of nursing action and select those actions which appear to be best suited to the problems, their origin and pathophysiology.

Nursing has, over the years, acquired many routine procedures. For some of these there is a well-established rationale. The efficacy of a few has been established by research. The professional nurse will constantly seek to review the basis of the prescription of nursing actions; some nurses may even test their effectiveness by research. The experienced nurse will internalise decisions about which nursing actions may be most appropriate. The student of nursing can gain a great deal by externalising the decisions she makes and writing down the rationale for her prescriptions of nursing action. This can often be a salutary experience and will stimulate further study.

The patient problems, the objectives or expected outcomes of nursing care and the nursing actions to achieve these outcomes are the core of the care plan, but it is not a static instrument. The nursing care of a patient is a dynamic and sometimes fast-moving undertaking. While the care is being carried out, there is need for review, reassessment and replanning; there also needs to be a statement about who should be carrying out the nursing actions, the environment in which the patient should be nursed, etc.; these factors are considered in the stage of implementation.

In summary, the care plan now has the following elements:

1. A nursing history for data collection.

2. Identification of patient problems (actual and potential) by assessment.

3. Objectives or expected outcomes of nursing care.

4. Nursing actions or the nursing care plan designed to achieve objectives.

The Kardex or other care plan document will accommodate these elements. The nursing history is usually on a separate sheet (see, for example, *Figure 4.5*). It is then useful if 'Patient problems', 'Expected outcomes' and 'Nursing actions' can be listed so that they can be seen alongside each other at a glance:

| Patient problems | Expected outcomes | Nursing actions (or nursing care plan) |
|---|---|---|
|  |  |  |

## Stage 4: Implementation

| Elements | Skills |
|---|---|
| Putting the plan into action. | Using technical and inter-personal skills in caring. Teaching. Counselling. Organising work. |

### 1. *Range of dependency*

The stage of implementing the care plan for an individual patient means very simply putting the plan into practice by carrying out the prescribed nursing actions. The degree of self-care the patient himself can maintain will have been assessed and the plan of care takes this into account, so that nursing actions deal with gradations of dependency in nursing care. In extreme cases when, for example, the patient is unconscious or is an infant, the nurse may have to take complete responsibility for all the daily living activities and become a substitute for self-care. Short of this, the patient may be able to sustain sometimes more, sometimes less, of the optimum quantity and quality of daily living activities, and the nurse acts as his help or assistant or agent in self-care. This means careful referral to the patient as to what he likes done and how he usually does it.

## 2. *Categories of nursing action*

There are different categories of nursing action. Manual skills are needed to give physical help and assistance, but psychological skills are also needed to give emotional support and help. The nurse may also use counselling skills or, where information is needed, communication and teaching skills. Learning to nurse and implement care plans means practising to become competent in all these skills. In many nursing situations they are, of course, employed in combination. Help in coping with pain, for instance, may call for physical measures, psychological support, counselling and information giving.

## 3. *Providing the environment for care*

A major aspect of care planning is in providing a suitable environment for the care of the patient. If the prescribed nursing activities indicate that the patient requires an intensity of nursing observation and activities, he should be positioned in the ward where these are possible. Reduced mobility may indicate that the position should be near sanitary annexes (promotion of continence as part of the care plan may not otherwise be achieved). Basic ward hygiene and the design of equipment all contribute to an environment in which the plan of care can be safely and effectively carried out. Regaining independence in dressing and eating may not be possible without adapted clothing and eating facilities. The psychological environment is always important but may be of the essence in long-term care for the elderly and mentally ill. Providing a suitable environment is, therefore, an integral part of implementing the total care plan for an individual patient.

## 4. *The organisation of nursing*

The nursing skills to be used in the care of a patient are identified in the nursing care plan. It also needs to indicate which nurses should be responsible for implementing the plan. This organisation of care has for many years been seen as a function of the ward sister or charge nurse: she/he made an assessment of needs, decided by the nursing care required, and deployed nursing staff to carry out the plan of care, usually by assigning them tasks. In practice, it is usually found that the emphasis on analysing individual needs and planning to meet these needs on an individual basis means that nurses using the nursing process adopt a more patient-oriented approach in deploying nursing staff. They use modified forms of patient allocation or team nursing. This change in method of staff deployment is not easy for nurses who are accustomed to task allocation.

In Chapter 8 one method of staff deployment is described, but whatever method is used certain principles are involved. A trained nurse should always be responsible for drawing up the plan of care and evaluating its outcome and revising it, if necessary. But as part of their training students need to be taught care planning and gain practice in the skill under supervision; the ward sister or charge nurse may, therefore, delegate care planning for some patients to another trained nurse in the team and the trained nurses may well supervise a student in care planning. As this happens, the role of the sister/charge nurse changes. Preferably she should always retain responsibility for the care plans of a few patients, but while she retains responsibility and accountability she may delegate planning for some patients to other trained staff. If she does this, she has an enhanced supervisory role. Similarly, the relationship with medical colleagues may change. This is described in Chapter 8.

The importance of a trained nurse, or a student under the supervision of a trained nurse carrying out the assessment, is stressed. In the ward described later in this book, this nurse is called the 'primary' nurse because she is primarily responsible for the care of the individual patient. She assesses his problems, plans his care and evaluates it. She retains accountability for his care throughout his stay. She will, however, often need assistance with implementing the care plan and carrying out the nursing actions she prescribes. While she is on duty, some nursing actions are best carried out by two nurses (e.g. lifting and bed-making); when she is off duty, the prescribed nursing actions need to be implemented. The primary or personal nurse needs therefore to have an associate nurse identified with her. After a spell off duty, the primary nurse needs to have a report on the progress of the patient, the outcomes of any care given and any indications that the plan of care should be changed. It is the primary nurse's role to see that the plan of care is implemented and reassessment and replanning carried out. In this way, the systematic plan is communicated to everyone involved in the care of the patient and erratic changes in care do not take place with shift change.

There is a clear line of responsibility and accountability for clinical care and its supervision, the ultimate responsibility resting with the sister or charge nurse to identify the primary and associate nurses for each patient. The implications of this are that the primary nurse will be able to give new detailed information to the consultant and other medical staff about any patient allocated to her. They, in turn, need to communicate with her about any diagnostic tests or aspects of treatment which might modify the care plan, and these need to be incorporated into the plan.

Nurses are usually responsible for co-ordinating all aspects of health care in the pattern of the patient's day. Whether primary nurses are identified or not, the responsibility for the care plan needs to rest with a clearly identified nurse who must take responsibility for implementation.

In summary, implementation involves:

1. Adjusting nursing action to the degree of dependence of the patient.
2. The use of different categories of nursing skill (manual, psychological, counselling, communicating and teaching) in carrying out prescribed nursing actions.
3. The provision of a suitable environment for care.
4. The organisation of nursing care by identification of the nurse with primary responsibility for the patient's assessment and care plan, and the identification of associate nurses to help in implementing the care plan.

## Stage 5: Evaluation

| Elements | Skills |
|---|---|
| Comparing actual outcomes with expected outcomes. Reassessment. | Assessment. |

The last stage in the process is evaluation; that is, evaluation of the care given. The major emphasis is placed on comparing actual patient outcomes with the stated expected outcomes. If the care plan has stated the objectives or expected outcomes clearly in terms of the changes one expects to see in the patient over a given period of time, then it is possible to assess whether these have been achieved. This is why a clear statement of expected outcomes is so important. Without it, evaluation of the effectiveness of nursing care becomes vague and subjective. Evaluation is a form of reassessment. The nursing care for a problem of reduced fluid intake for which the expected outcome was '$2\frac{1}{2}$ litres of fluid by mouth in 24 hours', can be evaluated by observing and recording the actual fluid intake over 24 hours.

Relief of pain can be evaluated by the patient's report of his subjective experience. Criteria for evaluation of nursing care are therefore aspects of patient behaviour:

1. What the patient says.
2. What the patient does.
3. How the patient looks.

They are the same aspects of his behaviour by which we first assessed he had a problem in self-care. The problem of 'inability to walk' is replaced by an 'ability to take three steps with assistance'; and 'inability to maintain personal hygiene' is replaced by 'ability to wash own face with assistance'. Assessing the effectiveness of nursing care in this way draws attention to the importance of having precise objectives and stating the time interval in which they should be achieved.

The written care plan thus needs a fourth column added; that is, 'Actual outcomes', 'Progress notes' or 'Evaluation'. Some would add to this a fifth column 'Date achieved' or 'Date (nursing action) discontinued'. Thus:

| Patient problems | Expected outcomes | Nursing actions | Progress (actual outcomes) | Date discontinued |
|---|---|---|---|---|
| | | | | |

The more clearly these columns can be seen together the better, although this calls for some skill in designing the layout of forms:

In summary, the nursing care plan has the following elements:

1. A nursing history by data collection.

2. Identification of patient problems (actual and potential) from the data by assessment.

3. Objectives or expected outcomes of nursing care.

4. Nursing actions or the nursing care plans to achieve objective.

5. Progress notes or actual outcomes (evaluation).

6. Date of discontinuation of nursing actions.

## *Non-achievement of objectives*

The objectives set may not always be achieved. There may be a number of reasons for this:

(a) The assessment was inadequate or inaccurate.

(b) The nursing actions prescribed were unsuitable, i.e. inappropriate or unrealistic.

(c) The nursing actions were not adequately implemented.

(d) The expected outcomes were not adequately perceived.

In other words, failure to achieve an objective calls for a review of each stage of the process and the effectiveness with which it has been carried out. The process becomes circular (see *Figure 3.2*) as the assessment, plan and implementation are reviewed, or it may be found that some new and intervening factor of which we had been unaware needs to be taken into the plan.

Evaluation by expected patient outcomes is thus a part of what is meant by a systematic use of the nursing process, but the review of each stage of the process is a way of evaluating nurse performance in each of the stages. It is professionally desirable for the nurse to be able to stand back from her performance and try to judge how adequate it is. The stages of the nursing process form a basis for the nurse reviewing her own performance (self-evaluation), or she can ask a colleague to evaluate her assessment, planning and action skills (peer evaluation). For purposes of registration or supervisory control, evaluation by a supervisor may be carried out using the nursing process. One useful strategy for peer evaluation is to have a colleague present the care plans for a patient to the ward staff. Such a discussion is held once a month in the nursing unit associated with the Department of Nursing at the Manchester Royal Infirmary. It is a useful learning experience to review together the adequacy with which patient problems have been identified, the inferences made from information and the effectiveness of the nursing actions prescribed.

Part II of this book describes the active use of the nursing process in our experience. For the sake of simplicity we have presented a view of the nursing process applied to patients in hospital. It is our opinion that the process is equally applicable in specialties such as district and psychiatric nursing, in midwifery and in health visiting. Certain changes of emphasis and techniques may be required, but the decision-making approach to planning can be adapted to all fields of nursing, midwifery and health visiting.

# Part II

# THE PRACTICE OF NURSING USING THE NURSING PROCESS

## Introduction

In Part I a framework for the practice of nursing and the use of the nursing process was outlined. In Part II the system developed in association with the Department of Nursing in the University of Manchester is described and the practical implications examined in greater depth.

A professorial nursing unit was established at the Manchester Royal Infirmary in 1976 to provide a clinical base for the University Department of Nursing. The stated objectives in establishing the unit were:

1. The establishment of a base for clinical practice for the Department of Nursing, giving it credibility in the eyes of students, medical and nursing staff and the public.
2. The establishment and evaluation of joint appointments between the National Health Service and the University Department so that the teaching of the department is based on realistic practice.
3. The testing of approaches to the management of nursing care taught in the department through, for example, the use of the nursing process.
4. Testing the 'interface' between medical and nursing practice in decision-making about care.
5. Providing a setting in which clinical methods can be tested.

In the Preface, reference was made to the two initial joint appointments, made with Health Service responsibility, of half time ward sister and charge nurse in a trauma ward. After an orientation period, changes in the organisation of nursing work (from job assignment to a patient-centred approach) and changes toward implementing the nursing process were made. Methods of assessment and recording were modified as experience was gained. After three years the joint appointments were moved to a new geriatric assessment ward where further developments were made. The chapters which follow draw on experience in both settings.

**4**

# Data Collection in Practice

We have found with experience that gathering information about the patient or taking the nursing history is best carried out in two stages:

1. The first stage nursing history is carried out shortly after the patient is admitted to hospital and provides enough information for the nurse to start looking after the patient. The information is gathered in (a) a relatively short and superficial interview with the patient and/or his relative or friend; (b) a systematic head-to-toe examination of the patient; and (c) an assessment of liability to bedsores using the Norton (1975) or Knoll (Blicharz, 1979) scores.
2. The second stage nursing history entails more detailed physical and psychological examination, and may include the use of more sophisticated tools in special problem areas, e.g. nutritional status.

## First stage nursing history

The general format of the first stage of the nursing history is shown in *Figure 4.1*. It has a number of headings (the major ones of which are given below), with spaces for the nurses to enter the details.

LIKES TO BE REFERRED TO AS:

This is an important piece of information to begin with. Not all elderly people like to be addressed by their first name or called 'Gran'. Children may have a pet name and not respond to their official name.

REASON FOR ADMISSION:

It is useful to know what the patient and his family see as the reason for his admission. This is not always the same as the medical reason for admission and should be checked against it.

WHAT PATIENT OR FAMILY UNDERSTANDS ABOUT HIS/HER CONDITION:

The patient or his family may have a very incomplete or even erroneous idea about his illness and the reason for his admission. For example, does he realise that he will be in hospital for a minimum of 14 weeks with a fractured femur; or does he know that he has cancer and is to have further cytotoxic

| Surname | Forename(s) |
|---|---|

**Address:**

**Next of Kin:**

**Date of Birth:**

**Age:**

**Relevant Tel. Nos.**

**Likes to be referred to as:**

**Date of Admission to Hospital:**

**Ward:**

**General Practitioner:**

**Reason for Admission:**

**Medical Diagnosis:**

**Consultant:**

**What Patient or Family understands about his/her condition:**

**Patient's and/or Family Reaction to Hospital Admission:**

**Home Conditions·**

*Figure 4.1*   First stage nursing history format

| History taken from | |
|---|---|
| LM782 | Record No. |

Meaningful Person in Life:                    Significant others/pets:

Community Resources (D.N.H.V., Social Worker, Meals on Wheels etc. . . .):

General Health History & Previous Hospital Admission:

Religious Practices or Beliefs Patient finds helpful:

Recreational Activities and Past/Present Work Life:

General Assessment on Admission:

*N.B.*  Note the name of the person who carried out the assessment and if patient or relative or both  involved

| Signature | Date |
|---|---|

**Figure 4.1**  continued

therapy? Whatever the patient's perceptions about his illness, they have important implications for the nurse's communications with him.

### PATIENT'S AND/OR FAMILY REACTION TO HOSPITAL ADMISSION:

It is useful to assess the patient's and/or family reaction to his admission. The patient may talk freely about his anxieties or he may be reluctant to talk and the anxieties remain unexposed. The patient may be unable to share even with his closest relatives the anxiety he feels. It is important that such situations should be taken into account in the care plan.

### HOME CONDITIONS:

Knowledge of the home environment is important when planning rehabilitation and discharge. For example, knowing that a cardiac patient lives in a high rise flat without a lift is important for planning purposes; outside toilets and steps may be a hazard to an elderly person, as may the adequacy of the heating system if, for example, it requires the patient to lift heavy hods of coal.

### MEANINGFUL PERSON IN LIFE:

Relatives, however close, are not necessarily the meaningful people in a person's life. They may live too far away to be involved in day-to-day contact or they may not wish to be involved. The most significant person in somebody's life may well be his next door neighbour, milkman or the local policeman. Many old people are unfortunately without meaningful friends, and their pet may be the most significant being in their lives. If this is so, the plan of care should take this into account.

### COMMUNITY RESOURCES:

Information about help from professional or voluntary services before admission may give some indication of the dependence of the patient and help in discharge planning.

### GENERAL HEALTH HISTORY AND PREVIOUS HOSPITAL ADMISSION:

At this stage of assessment it is useful to check on the present and previous health status. Information about allergies, chronic illnesses and drug regimes, such as insulin or steroids, is needed. It is useful to know if the patient has recently been in hospital and what his previous hospital experiences have been like.

### RELIGIOUS PRACTICES OR BELIEFS PATIENT FINDS HELPFUL:

In planning for the patient's spiritual needs it is more important to identify significant practices than a particular denomination. Illness often awakens or accentuates a spiritual need and nurses need to develop the skill of encouraging the patient to express his feelings and needs for certain spiritual observances such as having running water poured over his hands prior to meals, or setting apart certain times of the day for silence or prayer.

RECREATIONAL ACTIVITIES AND PAST/PRESENT WORK LIFE:

Knowledge of recreational activities such as the reading of books, magazines and papers, or listening to radio programmes and music, may prove useful in planning the patient's day to relieve boredom and inactivity, or in helping in the rehabilitation of a stroke patient or the patient recovering from a severe head injury.

Working life and general life-style may be permanently altered due to the effects of illness. In some cases the past work and life-style may contribute to or worsen illness.

GENERAL ASSESSMENT ON ADMISSION:

The first stage history should end with a brief description of the patient's physical and emotional state on admission. A systematic head-to-toe observation can be carried out using the Assessment Man (*Figure 4.2*). This helps to identify, for example, difficulty in breathing, poor peripheral circulation, skin condition, nutritional state, mobility, and sensory disturbances.

The baseline information is completed with recordings of temperature, pulse, respirations, blood pressure and weight. Liability to pressure sores is assessed using the Knoll Pharmaceutical Scale (*Figure 4.3*). The higher the patient scores in total on this scale, the more likely the risk of pressure sores developing.

Examples of first stage assessments are given in *Figures 4.4–4.6*.

# Second stage nursing history

The second stage nursing history entails more detailed physical and pyschological examination of the patient. This may be carried out at the same time or shortly after the first stage; it may also be used for regular up-dating and reassessment of the patient's condition and nursing problems. The content of this history is shown in *Figure 4.7*.

The two separate columns in the second stage history forms are headed 'History or usual condition' and 'Present condition/behaviour'. They are set out this way so as to identify problems with self-care and to assess how the patient is adapting.

Some nurses refer to the first column as history or usual condition when the patient is healthy at home, and to the second column as the present adaptation to ill health now that the patient is in hospital.

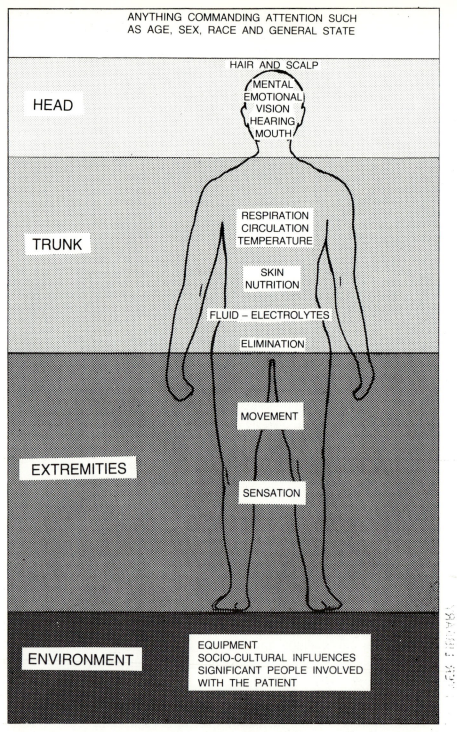

*Figure 4.2*   The Assessment Man — a head-to-toe guide to a patient's assessment on admission (after Wolff and Erickson, 1977)

| PARAMETERS | 0 | 1 | 2 | 3 | Score |
|---|---|---|---|---|---|
| General state of health | Good | Fair | Poor | Moribund | |
| Mental status | Alert | Lethargic | Semi-comatose | Comatose | |
| | | | Count These Conditions As Double: | | |
| Activity | Ambulatory | Needs help | Chairfast | Bedfast | |
| Mobility | Full | Limited | Very limited | Immobile | |
| Incontinence | None | Occasional | Usually of urine | Total of urine and feces | |
| Oral nutrition intake | Good | Fair | Poor | None | |
| Oral fluid intake | Good | Fair | Poor | None | |
| Predisposing diseases (Diabetes, neuropathies, vascular disease, anemias) | Absent | Slight | Moderate | Severe | |

The higher the score, the greater is the potential to develop decubitus ulcers. Patients with scores above [12] should be considered at risk.

**Figure 4.3**   The Knoll scale of liability to pressure sores (by courtesy of Knoll Pharmaceutical Co. New Jersey, 1977)

| | |
|---|---|
| Surname | Forename(s) |

Address:

Next of Kin:

Date of Birth:

Age:

Relevant Tel. Nos.

Likes to be referred to as:

Date of Admission to Hospital:

Ward:

General Practitioner:

Reason for Admission:

Medical Diagnosis:   From patient/family or medical/community nurse notes – brief details only if lengthy explanation given in medical notes.

Consultant:

What Patient or Family understands about his/her condition:

_____ Patient knows reasons for admission or _____

_____ relative/friend knows about medical condition. _____

_____ Some idea of what is wrong and possible prognosis. _____

Patient's and/or Family Reaction to Hospital Admission:

__ Expectations: _____ Pleased something is being done _____

__ Confused: _____ Anxious _____

__ Depressed: _____

Home Conditions:

__ Type of house/flat _____ Heated by (coal, gas, central heating) _____

__ Living alone _____

__ Potential difficulties on discharge (e.g. outside W.C. awkward—numerous stairs). _____

__ No shops in vicinity. _____

*Figure 4.4*   First stage nursing history — teaching prompt

| History taken from | |
|---|---|
| LM782  Record No. | |

**Meaningful Person in Life:**

Family/friends,
neighbours.

**Significant others/pets:**

Who does patient have close contact with?
Any pets (dog/bird, cat, other)?

**Community Resources (D.N.H.V., Social Worker, Meals on Wheels etc. . . .):**

Name of District Nurse, Health Visitor,
Social Worker.
Friends or helpers in local area near home.

**General Health History & Previous Hospital Admission:**

_____ Check medical notes. _____

_____ Note allergies (e.g. PENICILLIN). _____

_____ Chronic illnesses. _____

_____ Note if patient taking any drugs at present and, if so, that these have been brought in. _____

**Religious Practices or Beliefs Patient finds helpful:**

C/E Methodist, R/C, non-churchgoer, Agnostic, Atheist, believes in God.

**Recreational Activities and Past/Present Work Life:**
Hobbies    Job    Music (type)    Interests    Reads (type)
TV/Radio—Favourite programme

**General Assessment on Admission:**

_____ (see Assessment Man, Figure 4.2) _____

___ Brief details of patient's physical and emotional state on admission including skin _____

___ condition, conscious level, and any significant nursing observations. _____

___ Blood pressure  Temperature  Pulse  Respirations _____

___ Urinalysis  Bowel/Bladder function, and pain assessment _____

___ (Make note of any valuables/money brought into hospital) _____

_N.B._   Note the name of the person who carried out the assessment and if patient or relative or both  involved

| Signature | Date |
|---|---|

_Figure 4.4_    continued

| Can | John | |
|---|---|---|
| Surname | Forename(s) | |

**Address:** 7 Wellington Place,
Newholme, Lancashire

| Next of Kin: | | Date of Birth: 17·3·38 |
| | | Age: 42 years |
| | Wife | Relevant Tel. Nos. |
| Likes to be referred to as: | | |
| | John | 444 - 1311 |

| Date of Admission to Hospital: 3/6/80 | Ward: Trauma Unit |
|---|---|

**General Practitioner:** Dr. Stoke

**Reason for Admission:** "Had been celebrating with workmates, came home and fell backwards through a glass window into his garage at home." Landed on the roof of his car and rolled off onto the ground.

**Medical Diagnosis:** Fracture dislocation T12/L1

**Consultant:** Mr. Say

**What Patient or Family understands about his/her condition:**

Not sure of the extent of his injuries - says he feels "numb" below his waist.

**Patient's and/or Family Reaction to Hospital Admission:**

Very anxious about possible length of hospitalisation. Wife and children very upset at father's admission and reasons behind it.

**Home Conditions:**

Mortgaged dormer bungalow with central heating - bedrooms upstairs, large living cum dining room downstairs.

*Figure 4.5* First stage nursing history — example 1

History taken from

**By Nurse Castle from patient**

Record No. **4321**

Meaningful Person in Life:                     Significant others/pets:

Wife and 2 sons (1 15years and 1 18 years). Father who is alive and well.
2 sisters. 3 good workmates.

Community Resources (D.N.H.V., Social Worker, Meals on Wheels etc....):

Never needed any such resources before.

General Health History & Previous Hospital Admission:

Never had any major illnesses or health problems — never been aware of allergies to
anything.

Religious Practices or Beliefs Patient finds helpful:

Roman Catholic — goes to church regularly and would like visits while in hospital.

Recreational Activities and Past/Present Work Life: Works as a postman. Goes drinking with mates every Friday
and Sunday evenings. Enjoys gardening and watching football on T.V.

General Assessment on Admission: Admitted to ward from theatre following open reduction and fixation
of spine. General condition good, no signs of skin breakdown. No difficulty breathing when lying
flat on his side. Pulse rate and circulation good. Altered sensation below waistline — generally numb
and can feel pain and warmth when turned on right side. Difficulty moving both legs but can move
both feet up and down. Right stronger than left. Catheter in situ — may become constipated.
Oriented to time, place and person.

B.P. $\frac{110}{60}$   Pulse 72    Temp. 37°C Resps 20    Weight 168 lb

*N.B.*   Note the name of the person who carried out the assessment and if patient or relative or both
        involved

Signature   **R. Castle**                          Date

*Figure 4.5*   continued

| Arthur | Nancy |
|---|---|
| Surname | Forename(s) |

**Address:** 130 Coronation Road, Mossey Side, Manchester

| Next of Kin: | Date of Birth: 8·6·96 |
|---|---|
| Husband | Age: 83 years |
| | Relevant Tel. Nos. |
| Likes to be referred to as: "Nan" | 414 – 1113 (Neighbour – Mrs Smart) |

| Date of Admission to Hospital: 13·10·79 | Ward: G.1 |
|---|---|

**General Practitioner:** Dr. Ban  –  414 - 7721

**Reason for Admission:** For rehabilitation and promotion of self-care and continence. Only able to sit on sofa all day at home. Use sign language. Deaf - speech difficulty - can lip read.

**Medical Diagnosis:** Heart failure   Arthritis

**Consultant:** Dr. See

**What Patient or Family understands about his/her condition:**

Appears to appreciate and know the difficulties she has with her arthritis but does not seem to accept incontinence as a problem.

**Patient's and/or Family Reaction to Hospital Admission:**

When visited at home was reluctant to come into hospital. Only accepted the offer on the understanding that her husband would come in as well.

**Home Conditions:**

Pre-war back-to-back terraced house, no garden, outside toilet isn't used. Commode in living room. Doesn't use back room downstairs. Large gas fire, sofa, T.V. Doesn't cook  next door neighbour comes in.

*Figure 4.6*   First stage nursing history — example 2

| History taken from | |
|---|---|
| Patient and husband by Nurse Camille | |
| | Record No.  11211 |

| Meaningful Person in Life: | Significant others/pets: |
|---|---|
| Husband - Harry | Neighbour - Mrs Smart (414 - 1113) |
| (daughter died aged 11 years) | |

Community Resources (D.N.H.V., Social Worker, Meals on Wheels etc. . . .):

District nurse Johnson - 414 - 2111 and colleagues
Meals on wheels - daily and at weekends
Social work   Mr King - (deaf specialist) 221 - 1132

General Health History & Previous Hospital Admission:

May 1969  R leg ulcer - Whitworth Hospital
Allergic to strapping - not sure of make
Arthritis (Rheumatoid) 20 years   Heart failure 6 years

Religious Practices or Beliefs Patient finds helpful: Church of England. Says she is reluctant to see any
clergy now, since she has not been to church for years

Recreational Activities and Past/Present Work Life: Worked as a machinist in a shirt factory. Likes T.V.
and women's magazines when she can get them. Likes flowers and bright colours.

General Assessment on Admission:

Dehydrated, frail and ill-looking lady with brittle nails, poor personal hygiene and dry mouth
with damaged dentures. Sleeps always 4 pillows in the upright position. Urinary rash - signs of
skin breakdown on both buttocks, dry scaly skin on both legs. Communicates by sign
language and words - no sentences. 3cm x 3cm pressure sore. Superficial breakdown on
sacrum. Orientated to time, place and person.
Temp. 36·8°C Pulse 90  B.P. $\frac{160}{90}$   Weight 126 lb
Urinalysis  protein ++ Ketones ++
Nil else. Pressure sore potential high

*N.B.*  Note the name of the person who carried out the assessment and if patient or relative or both  involved

| Signature  G. Camille | Date 28/1/80 |
|---|---|

*Figure 4.6*   continued

| History or Usual Condition | Present Condition/Behaviour |
|---|---|
| (I) Basic Physiological Factors<br>(a) Activity/Movement<br>Use of aid, e.g. frame, walking stick, gait:<br>Ability to move in bed/chair.<br><br>(b) Rest/Sleep<br>Length, time, sedation.<br><br>(c) Nutrition<br>Appetite.<br>Eating habits – frequency, amount, variety.<br>Likes/dislikes.<br>Difficulties – dysphagia, anorexia.<br>Nausea/vomiting.<br>Malnutrition.<br>Weight.<br><br>(d) (Elimination/Continent State)<br>Bowels/bladder.<br>Difficulties–frequency.<br>Remedies.<br>Routine urine test.<br><br>(e) Fluids and Electrolytes<br>Amount, type, frequency.<br>Likes, dislikes.<br>Dehydration.<br>Condition of mouth and teeth.<br><br>(f) Breathing and Circulatory State<br>Respiratory difficulties, cyanosis, hypoxia, number of pillows needed, peripheral circulation.<br><br>(g) (1) Pain – degree, usual method of coping with this.<br>(2) Sensory disturbances.<br>(3) Speech.<br>(4) Hearing – aids.<br>(5) Vision – aids – spectacles.<br>(6) Temperature of skin.<br>(7) Smell.<br><br>(h) Skin Condition<br>Wounds, cuts, abrasions, ulcers, pressure area lesions, size, colour, location, quality of hair. | |

**Figure 4.7** Second stage nursing history — teaching prompt

| History or Usual Condition | Present Condition/Behaviour |
|---|---|
| (II) *Emotional State* <br> (a) *Perception of Health* <br> Patient's insight into his health state and illness. Any awareness of imminent death, chronic illness or body image disturbance. <br><br> (b) *Conversational Ability* <br> Alert, orientated to time, place and person. Able to express and communicate his feelings and wishes. Vague, unwilling to communicate. Short term or long term memory loss. <br><br> (c) *Reaction to being a Patient* (in hospital) and being too dependent upon others. Level of interdependence. <br> Too dependent? <br> Too independent? <br> Knows when to seek nursing aid. <br><br> (d) *Significant Non-verbal Gestures* <br> Looks away, watches carefully, agitated, frowns, fumbles, bites nails, sits quietly, ruminates. <br><br> (e) *Usual Reactions to Stressful Events* <br> Ways of coping with problems in lifetime. Usual physical and emotional reactions to situations such as loss, pressure at work, pressure and stress at home, financial problems, injuries and past illnesses. <br><br> (f) *Observable Behaviour and Mood Swings* <br> Is the patient's behaviour appropriate to situation: <br><br> Co-operative    Anxious <br> Withdrawn     Calm <br> Irritable         Confused <br> Aggressive | |

**Figure 4.7**  continued

By carefully following the criteria listed under the assessment factors, a much clearer picture of the patient's progress, and his usual functioning prior to his present health state, is gained. For example:

| USUAL CONDITION | PRESENT CONDITION |
|---|---|
| *(a) Activity/Movement* | |
| Prior to present illness — used to walk down the street to shops with aid of walking stick. | Now only able to walk the length of the ward with a walking frame. |
| *(b) Rest/Sleep* | |
| Usually went to bed at 10 p.m. and read until midnight. Woke once during the night, usually to micturate. Got up at 6.30 a.m., washed, and breakfasted at 7.30 approx. Dozed in chair for about an hour in the afternoon. | Having difficulty in sleeping more than 2-4 hours; finds he wakes at 4 a.m. and unable to get back to sleep. Afternoon naps are shorter than he would like. |
| *(c) Emotional state* | |
| Usually able to concentrate and read several books a week. | Now finds difficulty in doing this. |

When taking a second stage history the patient's description of his life-style and problems should be backed up with more concrete and objective evidence gained by observation and physical assessment. Added to this information, the findings of the doctor and other health-care workers may be relevant. Results of special tests, X-rays and routine medical investigations may play a direct part in influencing the nursing care plan.

Eight basic physiological factors are listed and six aspects of emotional state are listed in the second stage history form (*Figure 4.7*). These are offered as suggestions and can be expanded and explored in greater depth with more sophisticated tools. Examples of these latter aids are:

1. The Parker M5 Continence Chart (*Figure 4.8*).

2. The Nutritional Status form (*Figure 4.9*).

3. The Glasgow Coma Scale for recording level of consciousness (*Figure 4.10*).

4. The Mental Confusion Scale (see Appendix II).

UNIVERSITY OF MANCHESTER – DEPARTMENT OF NURSING

PROFESSORIAL NURSING UNIT – THE PARKER M5 CONTINENCE CHART

■ – Continent asked for aid (bedpan, urinal, commode toilet)
▲ – Continent only when offered aid (bedpan, urinal, commode toilet)
O – Aid given same not used
R – Aid offered but refused

U – Incontinent of urine
F – Incontinent of faeces
✓ – Dry
X – Damp/Dribble

| Date | Morning | | | Afternoon | | | | | | Evening | | | | | Night | | | | | | | | | COMMENTS |
|---|---|---|---|---|---|---|---|---|---|---|---|---|---|---|---|---|---|---|---|---|---|---|---|---|
| | 9 | 10 | 11 | 12 | 1 | 2 | 3 | 4 | 5 | 6 | 7 | 8 | 9 | 10 | 11 | 12 | 1 | 2 | 3 | 4 | 5 | 6 | 7 | 8 | |

*Figure 4.8*　Parker M5 continence assessment chart—for plotting the progress and success of the measures used to promote continence

Take a dietary history from the patient, listing the foods he/she would normally eat at home.

*Sample Daily Menu Pattern*

| *Breakfast* | *Mid-Morning* | *Lunch* | *Mid-Afternoon* | *Evening Meal* | *Bedtime* |
| --- | --- | --- | --- | --- | --- |

Does the patient realise the importance of eating a balanced diet?
Has the patient a good appetite?
What are the patient's likes or dislikes?
What does the patient weigh?
What is his/her 'ideal' weight?
What is the patient's height approximately?
Do you consider the patient to be overweight/underweight?
Is the patient active?
Who does the cooking and shopping?
Has the patient any dentures?
What is the condition of the mouth and teeth?
Has the patient any feeding difficulties (dysphagia, anorexia, nausea or vomiting)
Does the patient have a tendency to be constipated?
Does the patient take adequate fluids?

*Nutrients which May be at Risk in the Elderly*
Calcium and Vitamin D
Iron
Vitamin C

*Do You Consider the Patient to be Eating a Balanced Diet?*
Comment fully

**Figure 4.9**  Nutritional status — teaching prompt

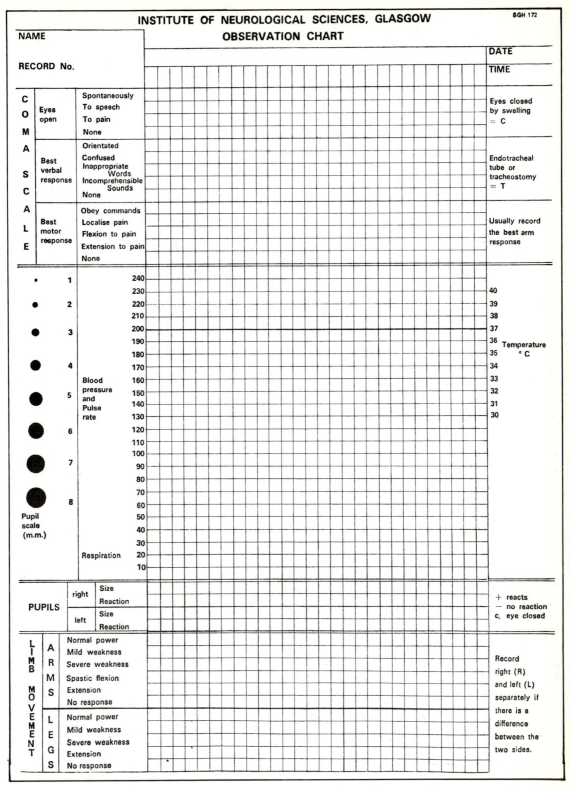

***Figure 4.10*** Glasgow coma scale — for recording level of consciousness (by courtesy of Professor G. Teasdale and the Editor of the *Nursing Times*)

## Process recordings

The patient may have problems in the areas of communications and interpersonal relationships. Process recordings can be a useful tool for assessing these.

Larkin and Backer (1977) point out: 'a process recording is a written description by the nurse of the verbal and non-verbal responses which occur between her and the patient.'

Process recordings usually consist of two parts: (a) a detailed recording and description of the verbal and non-verbal behaviour recorded during the interview, and (b) an analysis of interpretation of the meaning and significance of the recorded behaviour.

Process recordings will not only help in psychological assessment of patients, but will help the nurse to learn more about her own reactions.

# 5

# The Skills of Data Collection in Practice

## Interviewing

### *Before taking the nursing history*

It is important, before taking any information from the patient or his relatives and friends, to make sure that they are greeted in a polite and friendly manner. First impressions usually set the scene for how people will react later. The way an individual is greeted can affect both his attitude and frame of mind when he is interviewed.

For the patient, the stress of being admitted to hospital does not necessarily begin when he enters the ward. It may develop when he is at home following a visit by a consultant physician, or after a visit to the outpatients' department.

Other events which may have influenced the patient and his friends and relatives may have been the way the ambulance men have treated them, the hospital receptionist's attitude, or the hospital porter's behaviour on the way up to the ward.

On receiving a patient into the ward, it is important to allow for the anxieties and events which may have unsettled him, and which may upset the free, open and relaxed conversation which is essential for a successful nursing history interview. Greeting a patient in a wheel chair or on a stretcher by talking first of all to the porters or relatives who have accompanied him will not help him to feel you are interested in him as a person. For example, a paraplegic patient once related how dejected he felt when he was out with his wife in his wheel chair and people ignored him and asked his wife how he was.

It is important to let the patient know that he is expected and welcome, and to address him by name. For example, do not greet a patient by the organ or part of his body which is causing the problem: 'Oh hello, you must be the man with the leg!'

Patients who are kept waiting in a draughty corridor while someone prepares a bed for them will not be in the right frame of mind to start an interview.

If a short wait is unavoidable, then the area set aside for this should not be a gloomy part of the corridor. Comfortable chairs should be provided and information given as to the whereabouts of the nearest lavatories and facilities for a cup of tea. Bare walls and lack of decor suggest an institutionalised atmosphere. A safe rule is to treat new patients and visitors as one would treat a visitor in one's own home.

Talking with the patient and obtaining his nursing history are usually the first and often the most important parts of establishing a relationship and developing a more personalised approach to his nursing care.

## Preparation immediately prior to taking the nursing history

Before starting an interview, quickly review any previous source of inform- ation such as old nursing notes and the patient's medical records. Be careful, however, that such information does not condition the communication with the patient and prevent new approaches and ideas.

The following factors are important:

1. The setting for the interview should be private and as quiet as possible.

2. Both the nurse interviewer and interviewee should be comfortably positioned. The distance the nurse sits from the patient should not be too close or too far, and if possible she should try to avoid sitting behind a desk or bright light or peering over some form of barrier such as a cot side.

3. Interruptions should be minimised.

4. The nurse interviewer should be able to see the time.

5. The nurse interviewer should decide whether to use a checklist or questionnaire in front of the patient, and how to record the information.

Standard questions about age, address, religion, etc., should not be repeated if information is already available and a reliable and efficient clerk has filled in a comprehensive admission slip.

## Starting the interview

Some people feel more comfortable if you shake hands on first meeting them, so bear this in mind when you introduce yourself and explain the purpose of the interview. For example: 'Hello! Welcome to M5 ward! I am Nurse X. I will be responsible for looking after you during your stay in hospital. On this ward we allocate one nurse to each patient so that the care we give is more individual. Other nurses will, of course, help me in caring for you and you may ask any nurse for help, but I shall be mainly responsible for your nursing care. So that I can plan your nursing care, may I please ask you some questions about yourself?'

The content of the nursing history sheet (see *Figure 4.1*) contains a list of headings with a space below. Starting at any point on this sheet, you can think of appropriate questions and fill in the information, developing questions according to how comfortable the patient appears in answering them.

For example, a patient may have been brought into hospital by a neighbour; this would give you the chance to open your interview by finding out who is the most meaningful person in his life: 'I see that Mrs. Jones, your neighbour, brought you in; is this because you live alone?'

Alternatively, you may feel it better to begin the interview with a more generalised question, such as 'What brings you into hospital?' or 'What seems to be your present trouble?' Whichever question you start with, try to encourage the patient to enlarge or amplify his reply by saying something like, 'Tell me more about that'.

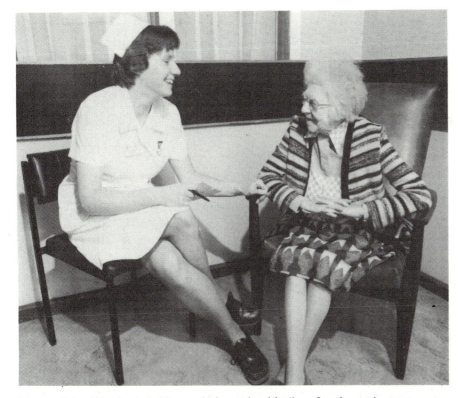

*Figure 5.1*    'The interviewing technique should allow for the patient to express his/her feelings spontaneously'

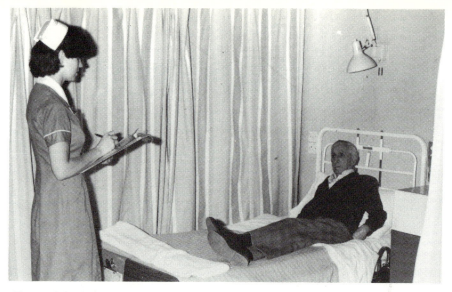

***Figure 5.2***   'The wrong technique — too threatening'

As the patient continues to respond you will pick up some type of 'thread' to his replies, and eventually you should be able to direct and gain the required answers to the headings shown on the history sheet.

Sometimes, however, not all the information outlined on the nursing history sheet can be obtained. A patient may, for example, be slightly confused.

The interviewing technique should allow for the patient to express his feelings spontaneously (*Figure 5.1*), which requires gaining the skill of listening and allowing the patient to talk, and knowing when to intervene and direct the patient on to a new subject. *Figure 5.2* illustrates the wrong technique — in this instance the interview is too threatening.

Some of the methods you can use to help and guide the patient without diverting him too much are classified according to Bates (1979), as follows:

(i)   *Facilitation:* This means saying very little except simple phrases such as 'Yes I see', 'Go on', or 'Then what?' Silence itself, used appropriately with non-verbal gestures, can encourage the patient to talk.

(ii)   *Reflection:* This consists of repeating certain phrases and words which the patient has used in describing what happened and which encourage him to carry on. For example:

Patient:   'The district nurse used to dress it.'
Nurse:     'Dress it?'
Patient:   'Yes, daily with Eusol solution.'

(iii) *Clarification:* The patient is using words which are ambiguous or unclear; therefore, you ask what he means by that phrase or word. For example:

Patient:  'I feel vexed with myself.'
Nurse:    'What do you mean by vexed?'
Patient:  'I mean . . . .'

(iv) *Empathic responses:* The patient expresses, with or without words, feelings about which he is embarrassed, ashamed or reticent. The nurse responds in a way that conveys sympathy and understanding so that the patient feels secure and encouraged to continue with his story. Examples of empathic responses are: 'That must have upset you', 'How difficult it must have been for you'. Non-verbal empathic responses can also be used; for example, offering a handkerchief, or placing your hand on the patient's arm.

(v) *Confrontation:* If you notice that the patient is trying to cover up his feelings or not acknowledging that he is angry, depressed or suffering from anxiety, you may feel it is best to confront him with your observations. This method is particularly helpful when faced with a patient who gives you an inconsistent history.

(vi) *Interpretation:* Interpretation goes a little further than confrontation and means that you make an inference about the patient rather than just a simple observation. For example:

Nurse:    'From what you have said, I would say that you are very angry about having to come to this ward.' (Be careful when using this technique or you may make the wrong inference and suggest something which may upset the patient.)

(vii) *Direct questions about feelings:* This means asking the patient straight, simple questions about how he feels or felt about something.

Eliciting the patient's feelings may well be crucial to understanding his illness and planning his nursing care. It is important, therefore, to encourage the patient to be involved in his future care by explaining the purpose of writing down his information and using it as a baseline or blueprint for future nursing actions. Example: 'Now that we have identified some of your problems, let us try to work out together how we can, as nurses, help you.'

If the patient is unconscious, confused, disorientated, or incapable of being interviewed on admission, then it is important that the nurse interviews the most appropriate person who will be able to help. Whoever this person may be, it is important to explain exactly why the information is needed and what will be done with it.

### Patient involvement

1. It has often been stated that the difference between frustration and despair may be the degree to which an individual feels he has some control over matters affecting him and his life. Involving the patient whenever possible is an essential factor of the nursing process approach.

2. The reasons for involving the patient are that he has the right to know what is going to happen to himself. He is more likely to co-operate and respond to his nursing care plan. Involvement helps relieve stress and anxieties, preserving the patient's sense of dignity and integrity and developing the relationship with his nurse.

3. Although the patient is perhaps the only one who truly knows what he feels he needs help with, it is essential not to forget the important and therapeutic role which relatives and close friends of the patient can play.

4. Involvement therefore includes encouraging relatives and close friends of the patient (i.e. 'significant others') to help the patient wherever and whenever possible.

5. Ways in which involvement can be encouraged are by seeking the patient's, or his significant others', views and thoughts when taking the nursing history and interviewing.

6. Included in the first stage nursing history are some suggestions for this. For example, 'What the patient or family understands about his/her condition.' When the assessment data has been collected the patient should be involved, if possible, in the statement and identification of his problems on the nursing care plan. Sitting down and going through the problem list with the patient can be very valuable in clarifying and communicating his problems and proposed nursing actions.

7. Involvement of the patient and his significant others should be encouraged to continue throughout hospitalisation and subsequent rehabilitation. The nurse should always be looking for ways in which this goal can be achieved. Helping with feeding, washing, walking and diversional therapy are some examples.

8. Finally, the patient's and significant others' views should be sought either at the end of certain nursing actions (*Figure 5.3*), for discussion at report hand-over time, or at evaluation conferences.

# Observation

Observation is a descriptive act which is accomplished by using the five senses: sight, smell, touch, taste and hearing. A point to bear in mind when writing nursing records is always to record descriptions of what you find, but not conclusions. One simple rule is to ask yourself the following question

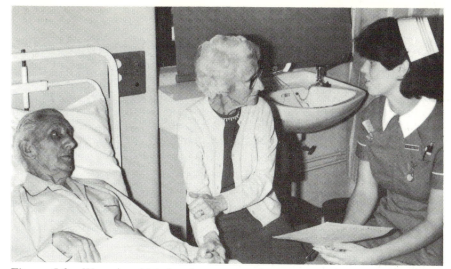

***Figure 5.3***  Ways in which involvement can be encouraged are by seeking 'the patient's and significant others' views, either at the end of certain nursing actions . . . or at evaluation conferences'

when you have completed your notes: 'Did I see, smell, touch, taste or hear what I have just written?' If your answer to this question is 'No' to all of the above five, then you have written a conclusion and not an observation. Likewise, if your answer is 'Yes' to all of the five, then you have written an observation.

The first stage history includes a systematic head-to-toe examination of the patient. The second stage history involves further examination of the factors listed. For example, the condition of the patient's hair/scalp, teeth, oral mucosa, movement of the chest, abdominal distension, obesity, muscle tone and mass, joint range, colour, texture and appearance of the skin and nails are observed.

Other factors to look out for are the patient's significant non-verbal gestures, such as use of eye contact, posture and manner of dressing. Evidence of oedema, lesions, skin breakdown, haemorrhage, pain and trauma should be noted.

When gathering information about the patient's family or close friends, observe the way they are acting towards the patient when they visit. If possible, contact the district nurse, health visitor or social worker if they have been involved with the family.

A visit to the patient's home can help in understanding the problems with which the patient may be faced on discharge. The neighbourhood, the physical appearance of the home, situation of the toilet, height of the bed, type of chairs, method of heating, access to rooms, number of stairs, bathing and cooking facilities — all may be relevant to his rehabilitation.

If it is possible, there is value in making this visit with the district nurse.

# Listening

Another very important and often underestimated means of observation is listening. Knowing how to listen involves channelling one's attention, concentrating on both the patient's verbal and non-verbal messages and shutting out external noise and distractions. If something is on your mind it may be very difficult to sit and carefully analyse what it is the patient is trying to communicate to you. Poor acoustics, noise, room temperature, ventilation and decor also have an effect. Irritating mannerisms or problems in speaking clearly may further distract the listener. Every now and then it is useful to review and summarise the points being made by the patient. One final point to remember, when listening to a patient, is to question the link between what the patient is saying and how he is acting.

## *Difficult situations*

There is no doubt that, however well your assessment skills develop, you will eventually come across some difficult situations. We have found the Bates (1979) special problems list to be helpful for considering the various types of difficulties:

(i)    *Anxiety:* Often expressed by the patient in the way he fidgets, sighs, sweats, trembles, sits tensely or finds it difficult to speak or relax. If you feel that this is happening, try to encourage the patient to talk about his feelings.

(ii)    *Anger and hostility:* Some patients may react angrily towards you because they may see you as a symbol of all that is wrong. Try not to react by getting angry yourself, allow the patient to ventilate his feelings and then seek a rational solution. Do not take sides with the patient against another colleague or part of the hospital, and do not rush off for a 'strong arm' or a psychiatrist.
Finally, it is important that you never promise things which you cannot carry out; for example, sending for a relative whom you know is unable to come.

(iii)    *Blind patients:* It is especially important when meeting a blind person to announce that you are with them, who you are and what you are doing. Touching the patient may help to establish contact and if you are distracted then inform the patient of what is happening.

(iv)    *Confusional behaviour:* Sometimes you may be halfway through an interview when you find out that the patient is contradicting himself. On the other hand, you may find that the patient is not answering your questions clearly and appears distant or aloof. If you are alert to this, you can switch your attention to some of the factors in the psychological assessment.

(v)  *Crying:* Like anger, crying should not be suppressed, as in most cases it is an important indicator of the patient's emotional response. The offer of a tissue, a supportive remark such as 'It's good to get it out', and placing a hand on the patient's arm, will help. When the patient has finished crying, he will probably feel better and capable of continuing the discussion.

(vi)  *Depression:* You may identify this in a patient who complains of tiredness, weight loss, insomnia and mysterious aches and pains. Careful questioning will help you with this situation.

(vii)  *Deafness:* Handwritten questions and answers may be the main solution. But be aware of non-verbal communications and lip-reading.

(viii)  *Fatally ill patients:* Often it is our own feelings and reactions which hinder the way we approach the fatally ill or dying patient. Be alert to the patient's feelings and to cues that he wants to talk about them. Try and make openings for the patient and explore those needs or problems he is having difficulty with. For example, 'I wonder if coming into hospital for this treatment is very upsetting for you?'

(ix)  *Language barriers:* The best solution in this situation is to find an interpretor or use drawings and non-verbal techniques. If you use an interpretor, explain to him the goals and purpose of your questions and make them short and to the point.

(x)  *Over-talkative patients:* This can be a particularly difficult problem when you have limited time in which to complete your assessment. Bates (1979) gives us four possible techniques of dealing with this situation:

  (a)  Lower your own goals and accept a less comprehensive history.

  (b)  Give the patient free rein for 5–10 minutes and weigh up the situation.

  (c)  Try to focus his account on what you judge to be the most important.

  (d)  Do not let your impatience show.

(xi)  *Patients with limited intelligence and literacy problems:* Although you can usually gain a fairly adequate history from these patients, beware that you do not overlook their limitations; for example, giving them instructions they cannot understand. Some patients with problems of reading may not easily admit it.

(xii) *Responding to patients' questions:* Patients usually seek simple factual information and it is important not to use medical jargon or go into long complicated accounts of what is happening to them. Remember, medical staff should give medical information and nurses should give the patient information about the nursing care aspects of his treatment. When you do not know the answer to a patient's direct question, it is usually best to be honest about it and say so, but do add that you will try to find out. Clearly acknowledging your status as a student may help you out of many awkward situations.

(xiii) *Silence:* Silences have many meanings and many uses. It is important to be aware of the patient's non-verbal actions during periods of silence and confront him carefully for the meaning of his actions; for example, 'You seem to be having difficulty talking about this?' Sometimes silence occurs when an interviewer asks too many direct questions in a rapid sequence or has offended or upset the interviewee.

(xiv) *Sexually attractive or seductive patients:* If you become aware of such feelings, accept them as normal human responses and try to prevent them from affecting your behaviour and professional standing. When it does happen, try to question yourself as to the image you are portraying and the way you are approaching your patients.

(xv) *Patients with multiple problems:* If you come across a patient who seems to have every problem under the sun, direct your interview into a psychosocial assessment, as the patient may have a serious emotional problem. On the other hand, it may be better to refer the patient to a trained nurse who is more skilled in this area.

# Completing the nursing history

Unfortunately, some patients are either totally or partially unable to contribute to the nursing history being carried out by the nurse. For this reason, and because we also believe that it is important to encourage family and friend involvement in nursing care, their help is sought. A spouse, for example, may be able to clarify certain areas of discrepancy in the information about the patient. It is important to keep this data in confidence, and only involve them when the patient approves and they are willing to co-operate.

The principles we have outlined, with regard to interviewing and collecting information from the patient, apply in conversations with relatives and friends.

## *Points to note when taking a nursing history and assessing a patient*

1. The object of taking a nursing history is to find out information about the patient, and how much the patient knows about the reasons why he is in hospital.

2. More information will be forthcoming from patients, relatives and friends if they are encouraged to talk freely about themselves. A long stream of questions may lead to short, abrupt answers. For example:

   Nurse:    'Have you been in hospital before, Mrs Smith?'
   Patient:  'Yes.'
   Nurse:    'Was this upsetting for you?'
   Patient:  'Yes, it was.'
   Nurse:    'What upset you?'
   Patient:  'I don't know.'
   Nurse:    'Don't you like hospitals?'
   Patient:  'No.'

An alternative, more open and simple question may be: 'What have been your previous experiences of nursing care in hospital?'

3. Be aware of non-verbal cues from patients and others when exploring areas of information which may be particularly sensitive. When a patient is reluctant to give information, do not push him for an answer; allow time for the patient to respond, but be prepared to shift the direction of your questions.

4. The use of pauses and silence can often help the patient to respond to questions.

5. Be sensitive to non-verbal cues, especially when the patient is becoming restless and tired. If you suspect this, then stop.

6. By encouraging patients to talk about themselves, relatively few questions need to be asked.

7. Only record relevant information about the patient which is essential to future nursing care.

8. When opening an interview, allow time for the patient to relax by discussing the weather or his journey to the hospital, or any other topic which will break the ice.

9. Always explain the purpose of the interview.

10. Discrepancies may be apparent when comparing information given to you by the patient and/or his relative/friend. There may be occasions

when you are not sure which is the true account. In this case, record quotations from both parties. For example:

Patient:    'I rarely suffer from dizzy spells, and have not had any during the last week or two.'
Daughter:  'I found him holding on to the table yesterday, and also last Sunday he fell over in the garden for no apparent reason.'

11.  If a patient wants to tell you something about his life which at first does not seem relevant, allow time for him to ventilate his feelings.

12.  One of the most useful phrases to use during an interview is, 'Tell me about . . . .'

13.  One of the more difficult aspects about interviewing patients is 'listening' to everything they have to say. The nurse's mind may be wandering on to other more pressing needs on the ward. To concentrate for more than 20 minutes on what a patient is saying is difficult.

14.  Be aware of your own reactions to the questions, and the answers you receive. Facial expressions may do a lot to encourage (or discourage) the patient.

15.  When interviewing, be careful not to:

(a)  Criticise.
(b)  Ask too many yes/no questions.
(c)  Ask leading questions which indicate the type of answer you expect.
(d)  Raise personal problems too soon.
(e)  Use 'gimmicky' questions which sound deep and searching.

16.  There is no straightforward answer to controlling a very talkative patient/relative/friend. One method is to interrupt at the end of a sentence and say something like: 'Thank you very much, that was interesting, but I wonder if you could give me an idea of what happened after that . . . .'

17.  In closing an interview, the nurse should:

(a)  Briefly summarise what she has learned about the patient.
(b)  Invite him to comment, add to or modify what she has written, or will be writing, about him.
(c)  Ask him if there is anything he would like to ask her.
(d)  Remind him that, although she has taken his relevant history now, there is no reason why further points could not be added at a later date.

18.  When the tensions of the formal interview are over, there are times when the patient/relative/friend may well tell you essential information about himself or the patient which is relevant to his nursing care.

19. Finally, only share with other colleagues (by writing precisely and concisely) that information about the patient which is relevant to his nursing care, and which the patient is willing for you to share. Other information, given in confidence, should be kept in confidence.

There is no doubt that interviewing and the assessment of patients requires practice and development of special skills. Role-play and the use of video machines can help the inexperienced nurse. Sitting in on an interview with a more experienced colleague can help, so long as you discuss the event afterwards. Even better, getting a more experienced interviewer to sit in with you and then discussing your technique afterwards may be more stressful but rewarding.

'The more you can learn about yourself, the better you will be at finding out information about the patient' (MacKenzie and McDonnell, 1975).

## *Time for taking the nursing history*

The time taken to gather all the information you need about a patient will vary considerably. It depends upon (a) the patient and his ability to communicate his needs and problems; (b) the skills of the assessor — the more experience you have had in carrying out this approach with patients, the more skilled you become; (c) the environment and atmosphere in which the communications are taking place; and (d) the needs of other patients — you should not ignore other patients in order to complete a detailed history of one particular patient.

There will be occasions when you will not have the time, or the opportunity, to explore all the areas of assessment in great detail. It is quite permissible to add this information at a later date. The essential assessment factors which should always be aimed for (except in extreme emergencies when the patient's life is threatened) are:

1. An introductory chat with the patient.

2. An idea of his emotional reactions and if he understands the reason for his admission.

3. General details such as full name, address, next of kin, age, significant past medical history and contact with nursing, telephone number for emergency use, current drugs and any allergies.

4. A head-to-toe systematic examination/observation of the patient to determine any existing or potential problem areas (see *Figure 4.2*).

5. A record of the patient's vital signs such as blood pressure, temperature, pulse, respirations, weight and urinalysis.

SURNAME                    FORENAME                    RECORD NO.

ADDRESS

Likes to be referred to as:

Date of admission:                          Ward:

Next of kin:                                Relevant tel. no.
                                            for emergency:

Date of birth:                              G.P.:
                                            (name & address)

What I understand about the reason for my admission:

Worries I have about my present state of health:

Significant illnesses or past hospitalisations I feel are important to tell you about:

Allergies:                                  Present medications:

Systematic head-to-toe review with aid of nurse (plus record of vital signs):

HEAD

TRUNK

                                            Blood pressure
                                            Temperature
                                            Pulse
                                            Respiratory
                                            Weight
                                            Urinalysis

EXTREMITIES

ENVIRONMENT

**Figure 5.4**    Nursing history format (see also *Figure 4.2* for head-to-toe assessment)

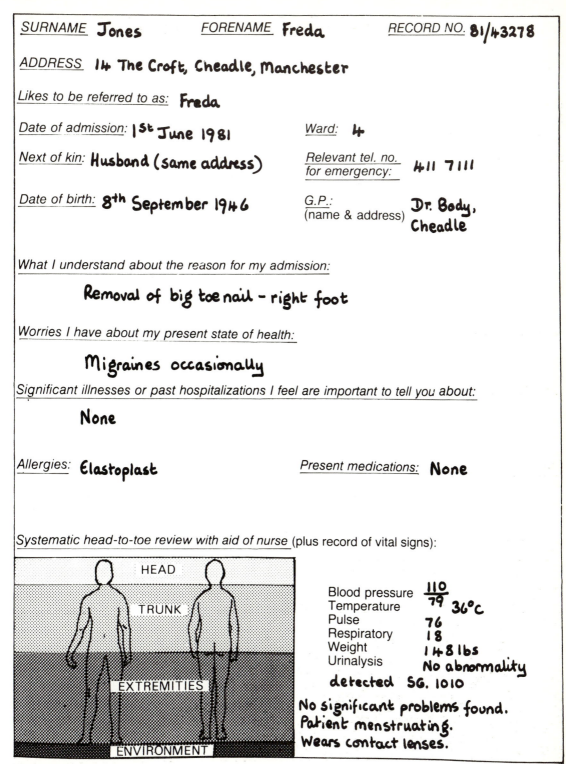

SURNAME  Jones        FORENAME  Freda        RECORD NO. 81/43278

ADDRESS  14 The Croft, Cheadle, Manchester

Likes to be referred to as:  Freda

Date of admission: 1st June 1981        Ward:  4

Next of kin: Husband (same address)    Relevant tel. no. for emergency: 411 7111

Date of birth: 8th September 1946      G.P.: (name & address)  Dr. Body, Cheadle

What I understand about the reason for my admission:

Removal of big toe nail - right foot

Worries I have about my present state of health:

Migraines occasionally

Significant illnesses or past hospitalizations I feel are important to tell you about:

None

Allergies: Elastoplast        Present medications: None

Systematic head-to-toe review with aid of nurse (plus record of vital signs):

HEAD

TRUNK

EXTREMITIES

ENVIRONMENT

Blood pressure  $\frac{110}{79}$ 36°C
Temperature
Pulse            76
Respiratory      18
Weight           148 lbs
Urinalysis       No abnormality detected SG. 1010

No significant problems found.
Patient menstruating.
Wears contact lenses.

**Figure 5.5**  Completed example of a nursing history

---

*STANDARD CARE PLAN* (would include):

Baseline observation

Fast from 6 a.m.

Remove dentures/contact lenses/other prosthesis

No make-up – clean skin

Shave operation site

Identity-band on right arm
      consent form completed
      notes & X-rays

Operation gown

Empty bladder

Security of valuables

Emotional support

---

*Figure 5.6*    Standard care plan and patient teaching guide

The gathering together of this baseline information should take no longer than 25-30 minutes. Remember, this is the total time and not necessarily the continuous time spent with the patient. Valuable time can be saved by interviewing and examining the patient at the same time as the doctor (see *Figure 9.10*). Co-operation and an understanding of each other's assessment goals are important for such a technique to be successful.

# The short-stay patient

The depth to which you should go with the nursing assessment of a patient depends upon the following:

1. What you are going to do with the information.

2. The extent to which you are going to help or care for the patient.

3. The complexity of the problems the patient is presenting.

In the case of a healthy individual being admitted to hospital for a relatively minor surgical or special test, the principles of the nursing process are followed but degree of depth and time taken varies. The same could be said of any nursing situation, for example in the community, when a patient may be visited only once, or in casualty when a patient is admitted for a few hours.

As an example of this type of approach, a female patient admitted for removal of a toe-nail, who will be in hospital for only 8 hours, is chosen.

The patient has been sent, prior to admission, a copy of the nursing history format to fill in (*Figure 5.4*). *Figure 5.5* shows a completed example of a nursing history. The patient will, in addition, have been sent a teaching guide as to the type of nursing care she will be receiving (*Figure 5.6*).

On the patient's admission to the ward, the nurse quickly goes over the completed nursing history, clarifying any areas which the patient did not understand. *Figure 5.7* illustrates what may be included in an individual care plan prior to an operation.

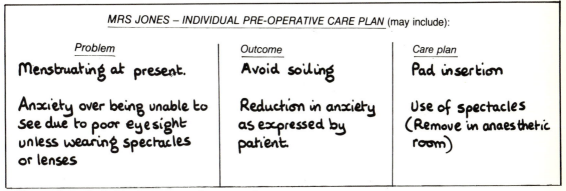

*MRS JONES – INDIVIDUAL PRE-OPERATIVE CARE PLAN* (may include):

| Problem | Outcome | Care plan |
|---|---|---|
| Menstruating at present. | Avoid soiling | Pad insertion |
| Anxiety over being unable to see due to poor eyesight unless wearing spectacles or lenses | Reduction in anxiety as expressed by patient. | Use of spectacles (Remove in anaesthetic room) |

**Figure 5.7** Individual pre-operative care plan

*STANDARD POST-OPERATIVE CARE PLAN*

Maintain clear airway

Half-hourly observations until stable vital signs

Check dressing

Check for any drainage tubes

Offer analgesics as required

Nil by mouth until 2 hours following return

Report progress in Kardex

Check urinary output

Sit patient up and give post-operative wash – help with dressing

Emotional support

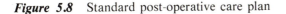

**Figure 5.8** Standard post-operative care plan

MRS JONES – INDIVIDUAL POST-OPERATIVE CARE PLAN

| Problem | Outcome | Care plan |
|---|---|---|
| Menstruating | Avoid soiling and personal embarrassment to patient | Change pad as required |
| Anxiety re vision | Patient expresses any anxiety | Use of spectacles on recovery from anaesthetic |

*Figure 5.9*   Individual post-operative care plan

Following the post-operative period, a standard care plan is followed (*Figure 5.8*) and any personal problems noted on the individual post-operative care plan (*Figure 5.9*).

On recovery, and prior to discharge, the nurse who has been looking after the patient should record any significant observations in the Kardex and the outcome of the nursing actions.

It may be possible to encourage the patient to express any feelings about the hospitalisation and nursing care received.

# 6

# Assessment in Practice

## Identifying problems

In the assessment stage, the information gathered in the nursing history is sorted and analysed for its significance so that the patient's problems with daily living activities are identified. The first example, given in the second stage history in Chapter 4, indicates a problem of decreasing ability to walk.

| USUAL CONDITION | PRESENT CONDITION |
|---|---|
| *(a) Activity/Movement* | |
| Used to walk down the street to shops with aid of walking stick. | Now only able to walk the length of the ward with a walking frame. |

The second example indicates a problem in preserving the normal sleep pattern:

| USUAL CONDITION | PRESENT CONDITION |
|---|---|
| *(b) Rest/Sleep* | |
| Usually went to bed at 10 p.m. and read until midnight. Woke once during the night, usually to micturate. Got up at 6.30 a.m., washed, and breakfasted at 7.30 approx. Dozed in chair for about an hour in the afternoon. | Having difficulty in sleeping more than 2–4 hours; finds he wakes at 4 a.m. and unable to get back to sleep. Afternoon naps are shorter than he would like. |

More information would be needed to make a precise statement of the problems; that is, to include the cause. It could, for example, be 'Disturbed sleep pattern due to change of environment and anxiety about admission'.

Having reviewed all the material in the nursing history, compared it with normal functioning for that patient, and made some judgements or inferences about its significance, the nurse can then make a list of patient problems, writing them down in order of priority.

For example, the nurse may have identified the following problems and placed them in an order of priority:

1. Maintenance of a clear airway.

2. Potential problem of pressure sores.

3. Maintenance of nutritional state and weight.

4. Help with personal hygiene and comfort.

5. Risk of sensory deprivation and isolation.

'A nursing problem is any condition or situation in which a patient requires help to maintain or regain a state of health, or to achieve a peaceful death' (Becknell and Smith, 1975).

The problem list is an itemisation of the problems which the nurse has discovered from the data collected from and about the patient. As Bower (1972) points out, problems arise when the patient, family or community

(a) cannot meet a need;

(b) need help in meeting a need;

(c) are not aware of an unmet need;

(d) have conflict of apparently equal needs;

(e) must choose from several alternative ways of meeting needs.

### Needs and problems

Following this approach, a problem exists when the patient for some reason cannot meet his need. Sometimes nurses have difficulty in sorting out what is a need and what may be a problem.

Very simply, all people have needs (e.g. breathing, feeding) with which usually they do not need nursing assistance. It is when there is a potential or actual breakdown in meeting a need that a potential problem or actual problem arises.

### Overt and covert problems

Some of the patient's problems are obvious and readily recognisable. Bower (1972) refers to these as *overt* problems. *Covert* problems, on the other hand, are those problems which are not so easily recognised or identified. The data collected in the nursing history needs to be carefully reviewed, or more sophisticated tools used (see *Figures 4.1–4.6*).

There is no doubt that many covert problems will become known to the nurse as she gets to know her patient through their daily interaction. This may be while she is finishing a bed bath or casually chatting to the patient when he may be waiting for a special medical test.

It is important, therefore, to encourge nurses to add this information to the nursing history and tell their colleagues about it.

# Actual and potential problems

Stating the patient's problems can be a complex task. It may be that the patient has no 'actual' problems demonstrated at the moment, but if you do not help him then problems may arise. Such possibilities are known as 'potential' problems.

When compiling the patient's problem list on the nursing care plan, it is important and very helpful to include both actual and potential problems, as shown below.

### *Example of actual and potential problems*

### *Actual patient problems*

1. Difficulty in feeding self, due to . . . .

2. Unable to stand without the assistance of two people.

3. Confused in time, place and person, due to . . . .

4. No insight into his illness, due to . . . .

5. Fear of anaesthetic, due to . . . .

### *Potential patient problems*

1. Potential problem of pressure sores, due to . . . .

2. Potential problem of dehydration, due to . . . .

3. Potential problem of confusion, due to . . . .

4. Potential problem of severe stress, due to . . . .

5. Potential problem of side-effects from drugs, due to . . . .

It may be helpful to add the reason for the actual or potential problem in your statement. Thus we may have, for example:

'Difficulty in feeding self, due to the effect of the cerebrovascular accident.'
'Potential problem of pressure sores, due to inability to turn himself.'
'Potential problem of confusion if patient moved to a new position in the ward.'

## Referring problems

Another difficulty which may arise is that the nurse may identify a problem which no nursing intervention can adequately deal with. For example, she might discover a difficult social problem which is better referred to the trained social worker.

It is important, therefore, for nurses to be encouraged to pass on information to others in the health-care team and act as co-ordinators of the patient's care.

## Patient's nursing problems *versus* medical diagnosis

One of the major difficulties when it comes to stating a patient's nursing problems is that many nurses get confused with the patient's medical diagnosis.

For example, a nurse may state that the patient has a chest infection instead of trying to find out what it is about the patient's chest infection that is causing him a problem which can be helped by nursing care. It may well be (a) difficulty in expectoration of sputum, or (b) difficulty in taking an adequate intake of fluid by mouth, or (c) difficulty in sitting upright in bed and performing deep breathing exercises.

Some problems, however, may relate to the patient's major medical symptoms, for example:

(a) pain;

(b) nausea and vomiting;

(c) dehydration;

(d) weakness in limbs;

(e) headaches due to intracranial pressure.

They may also be anticipated in certain medical situations, for example:

(i)   Slowing of the pulse, on Digoxin therapy. Potential problem of this falling below 60 beats per minute.

(ii)  Potential problem of bleeding if the patient is on anticoagulant therapy.

(iii) Post-operative pain.

Perhaps the only time when the patient's nursing problems are the same as his medical problems is in an emergency situation when the nurse's goals and actions are the same as the physician's; for example, in the case of cardiac arrest.

Even in situations where the nurse has insufficient information about the patient — for example, when the patient has been admitted in an unconscious state — the nurse should be trying to look at the situation from the patient's perspective, gradually piecing together scraps of information about the patient so that she treats him as an individual and identifies his problems.

When patients have difficulty in communicating the effects of an illness on them to nurses, there is a danger that they will be referred to by their medical diagnosis. For example: 'Where is the stroke we had in last night?'

# Statement of problems

The statement of a patient's problems on a care plan should be precise, concise, and to the point. Examples:

(i) *Incorrect way:* The patient has many bony prominences which appear to be areas where pressure sores could develop.

(i) *Correct way:* Potential problem of pressure sores, due to bony prominences.

(ii) *Incorrect way:* The patient is expressing considerable difficulty in keeping his 'cool' prior to the operation tomorrow.

(ii) *Correct way:* Expressed verbal anxiety due to operation tomorrow.

There is no doubt, as Bower (1972) points out, that 'a large part of the solution of a problem lies in knowing what it is you are trying to do'.

When writing down a problem it is sometimes a good idea to quote what the patient has said, as this sometimes conveys more feeling and individuality. Examples:

(i) Appears a little disorientated at times, occasionally asks: 'Is this a hotel I am in?'

(ii) Patient states that the pain 'is like a red hot poker' over his right eye.

Problem statements can also be descriptive in that they convey an account of what is happening to the patient under certain circumstances. Examples:

(i) Starts to cry when anybody mentions his wife.

(ii) Becomes constipated when bran is omitted from diet.

Some problems may relate to the aetiology of a patient's illness and some may be primarily physiological, pyschological or social in origin. They may be also a combination of any of these. For example, a patient may have an irritating skin condition which develops when he is emotionally upset in particular social circumstances.

To summarise the variety of ways problem statements can be made, Durand and Prince (1966) give us seven examples:

(i)   Descriptive.

(ii)  Aetiological.

(iii) Primarily physiological.
      Primarily psychological.
      Having aspects of both.

(iv)  Major medical symptom.

(v)   Anticipated in a certain medical condition.

(vi)  Distinct from the medical diagnosis or condition.

(vii) Medical diagnosis.

Sorting out patients' problems is rewarding and an essential exercise which requires careful thought and experience in nursing. It is important for the learner to check with a trained nurse that the problem list relates specifically to the patient and is not misleading or vague in its wording. There is a danger that what is written down is not the patient's problem but the problem the nurse is having in caring for the patient.

# 7

# Planning in Practice

Identifying and listing the patient's problems carefully and accurately is the objective of the assessment. The list of problems is the foundation on which the patient's nursing care plan is built. The nursing actions making up the plan must relate to each of the patient's problems and be designed with specific outcomes in mind.

There has been much discussion about what to include on a nursing care plan; the following example is one which has proved useful:

| Date identified | Patient's nursing problems | Expected outcome or goals/ objectives | Nursing care plan | Progress notes | (Actual outcomes) | Date resolved |
|---|---|---|---|---|---|---|
|  |  |  |  |  |  |  |

It is important to ask ourselves what are care plans supposed to do? First, they help to individualise the patient's nursing care by showing us what each patient requires. Secondly, they help us to sort out the priorities which we are having to deal with. Thirdly, they should be a clinical aid in communicating information to all the nursing staff and help other members of the health-care team to see what we are doing (*Figure 7.1*). Finally, they will help all the nursing staff who use them to develop a critical problem-solving approach to their patient's care.

## Expected outcomes

Before stating the plans of action to be taken by the nurse it is important to consider what we expect the patient to demonstrate as a result of nursing actions.

Therefore, the 'expected outcome' is a statement of what the nurse expects the patient will be able to achieve by a certain time or date; that is, it is a statement of expected patient behaviour. Many books on the nursing process refer to this as the objectives or goals of patient care.

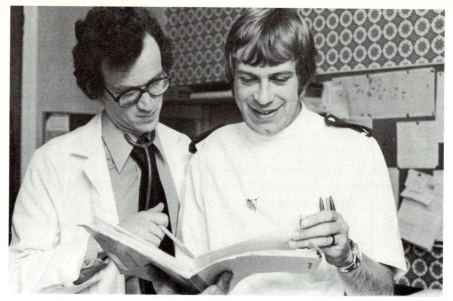

*Figure 7.1*   Care plans should be 'a clinical aid in communicating information to all the nursing staff and help other members of the health care team to see what we are doing'

The phrase 'expected outcome' was taken from Mayers (1978) and is the standard against which the success or failure of the nursing action is evaluated. It indicates that nursing objectives have been achieved.

When writing expected outcomes of care the nurse should consider the *subject* who is expected to demonstrate the behaviour. This may not be the patient. For example, the patient's problem is that he cannot inject his insulin because he is partially blind. The expected outcome, therefore, is that his wife (who is now the subject) should do this for him.

The second component in writing an expected outcome is that of *behaviour*. Only a verb should be used to express the expected behaviour; for example, verbs such as 'walk', 'drink', 'turn' and 'sit' are preferable to such terms as 'comfortable', 'satisfactory' and 'happy'.

Becknell and Smith (1975) also make an important point when they discourage the use of the words 'Patient will have . . . '. 'Will have' suggests that someone other than the patient or subject will be performing the behaviour. It is preferable to write 'Patient will move his bowels before noon' rather than 'Patient will have his bowels moved by noon'. Mayers (1978) suggests, as a practical guide for selecting the right sort of words and phrases, asking oneself: 'What do I *see* or *hear* that makes me believe that the patient has a problem?'

A third component to consider when writing expected outcomes is to state the *conditions* under which the behaviour is expected to be demonstrated. For example: 'The patient will walk to the table for his meals without assistance', or 'The patient will walk to the table for his meals using his walking frame'.

Stating the conditions under which a patient will perform certain actions helps nurses to realise exactly what they are trying to get the patient to do and what are the limitations.

Finally, the fourth component in writing expected outcomes is to state the *criterion* for the performance of a behaviour. For example, 'two hourly', 'twice a day' or 'once a week'.

Combining these four components, we have the following expected outcomes of care:

1. With the aid of a walking frame, the patient will walk to the table for his three main meals each day.

   Subject      = the patient.
   Behaviour   = will walk.
   Condition   = with a walking frame.
   Criterion    = to the table three times a day.

2. Will drink at least 1,500 mls. of fluid between 6.00 a.m. and 6.00 p.m. each day.

   Subject      = the patient.
   Behaviour   = will drink.
   Condition   = none.
   Criterion    = 1,500 mls. between 6.00 a.m. and 6.00 p.m.

From this second example it will be noted that no condition was stated, and in some cases it may be difficult to state the criterion under which an objective should be achieved. The most important factor, however, is for the nurse to attempt to write down at least a broad outcome of care and add a deadline date or time when she feels this will be achieved. As Mayers (1978) points out, 'an expected outcome is a statement of what the nurse expects to observe, hear or see demonstrated at a given point in time'.

| Date identified | Patient's problem | Expected outcome |
|---|---|---|
| 1st August 1980 | 1. Difficulty in breathing unless sitting upright in bed. Respiration = 40/min. | 1. Upright position in bed maintained by pillows and back rest. Respiration = 28/min. 2nd August 1980, 4.00 p.m. |

# The nursing care plan (prescription of nursing actions)

The third and final part of the planning process is the statement of the nurse's plan of action. This is sometimes referred to as the Nursing Orders or Prescription of Nursing Care and is defined by Becknell and Smith (1975) as:

'The prescription of specific methods or directions by which nursing care objectives are to be achieved and which assist in the management and/or solution of patients' nursing problems.'

In order for this part of the overall care plan to be useful, it is again important to stress that nursing orders should be written precisely, concisely and to the point.

It is important to number nursing actions on a care plan so that they correspond with the patient's nursing problem and expected outcomes. When the care plan is reviewed or updated, then a line is drawn through the problems and dated as discontinued if the problem has been resolved.

If it recurs at a later date, then the problem is entered again using another number. In this way the patient may have, say, 16 problems written down on a care plan, of which eight have been discontinued and one or two rewritten because they have recurred or changed in context.

When nursing orders have been stated, it is sometimes difficult to convey precisely the time for nursing actions. For example, to state that a patient should receive two hourly turns for pressure area care is inadequate unless you add when such turns should be carried out.

The nursing order must be a statement of the behaviour to be performed by the nurse and appropriate verbs of intent should be used; for example, 'walk', 'move', 'dress' and 'record'. There is a danger that vague words such as 'reassure' and 'encourage' will be interpreted in different ways.

When deciding upon a particular course of action it is important for the nurse to ask herself, 'What is the scientific evidence which supports the approach I am suggesting?' Questioning carefully the rationale behind proposed nursing actions will lead to more thoughtful and reliable nursing actions.

## *Plans for potential problems*

In certain cases some problems may be stated as 'potential' because they are likely to occur if something is not done by the nurse to prevent them. The nursing orders are written the same as they would be for other current problems, with the difference that these orders are geared toward preventing the onset of actual problems. Example:

1. Potential problem of pressure areas developing at . . . (name sites).
2. Potential problem of . . . (side-effects of drugs).
3. Potential problem of hypoglycaemic attacks.
4. Potential problem of injury due to blackouts.

## *Points to be aware of in planning the patient's care*

1. Each nursing problem identified should usually have its own objectives or expected outcome and plan of action. In some cases, however, some combined problems may have the same outcomes and plans.

2. Each problem and action should be dated and numbered when it is identified.

3. Write down first those problems which are a priority for immediate nursing action.

4. Try always to identify what the patient's problem is due to.

5. Always write care plans in ink.

6. If you make a mistake, put a line through what you have written and write 'error' over the top.

7. Always check care plans with a trained member of staff.

8. If you isolate problems for which you or any other trained nurse will be unable to do anything, then inform the patient and refer the problem — if the patient wishes it — to another agency or, if a medical problem, to a doctor.

9. Nursing care plans should demonstrate co-ordination with the over-all medical and general health-care plan for the patient.

10. Nursing prescriptions or proposed nursing action should be based on sound scientific knowledge and utilise appropriate research findings wherever possible.

11. Nursing objectives should form the basis for evaluation of care and, where possible, have stated deadlines.

12. Nursing plans should show the inter-relatedness of the psychosocial needs and the physiological needs of the patient.

13. Nursing plans should, where possible, reflect family involvement in the patient's nursing care.

14. Nursing plans should also reflect preparations for future transfer home.

15. In some instances, standard nursing care plans may be used where routine safety procedures are carried out.

16. Do not copy other patient's plans because the cases seem similar.

17. The statement of the patient's problem may be expressed in several ways:

    (a) Descriptive.
    (b) Aetiological.
    (c) Primarily physiological, primarily psychological, primarily social — or a combination of two or more of these.
    (d) Major medical symptom.
    (e) Anticipated in a certain medical diagnosis.
    (f) Distinct from the medical diagnosis.
    (g) The same as the medical diagnosis.

18. The care plan should also include those problems which concern the patient's family or other significant people as well as the patient's problems.

19. The patient's care plan should be up-dated and reviewed every day.

20. When problems are resolved, score a line through them, write 'resolved' across them and enter the date in the appropriate column.

21. If possible, review the problem list with the patient.

22. Do not forget to place the patient's name and unit number on the care plan and sign it.

23. Be precise, concise and to the point. Use expressive verbs and write possible objectives in behavioural terms.

24. Finally, when planning the patient's care, emphasis should be on arriving at common goals, especially if those of the patient and nurse are different.

### Types of care plan

There are three types of care plan: (1) problem-orientated care plan (*Figures 7.2* and *7.3*); (2) daily care plan – see below; (3) standard care plan.

## The daily care plan

In addition to the problem-orientated care plan described above, we have found that a more detailed and strict statement of what we hope the patient will be able to achieve at a specific time every day is helpful (*Figures 7.4* and *7.5*), particularly for patients who are very confused, disorientated and need some form of daily routine.

CARE PLAN

| Date Commenced | Patient's Nursing Problem | Expected Outcome | Nursing Care Plan | Tick when completed: Date/Time Discontinued | Tick when completed: Signature |
|---|---|---|---|---|---|
| | | | | | |
| | | | | | |
| | | | | | |
| | | | | | |
| | | | | | |
| | | | | | |
| | | | | | |
| | | | | | |
| | | | | | |
| | | | | | |
| | | | | | |
| | | | | | |
| | | | | | |
| | | | | | |
| | | | | | |
| | | | | | |
| | | | | | |
| | | | | | |
| | | | | | |
| | | | | | |
| | | | | | |
| | | | | | |
| | | | | | |
| | | | | | |
| | | | | | |
| | | | | | |
| | | | | | |

***Figure 7.2*** Problem-orientated care plan format

| Date Commenced | Patient's Nursing Problem | Expected Outcome | Nursing Care Plan | Tick when completed Date/Time Discontinued | Signature |
|---|---|---|---|---|---|
| | Precise/concise list of patient's nursing problems in order of priority, e.g.<br>1 Difficulty in breathing unless sitting upright in bed.<br>2 Potential problem of pressure sores due to inability to move freely in bed.<br>3 Difficulty in taking fluid by mouth. | Specific objectives which one is trying to achieve with this particular patient's problems.<br>1 Regular free and easy intake of air – no cyanosis.<br>2 Avoid skin breakdown at buttocks and elbows.<br>3 2½ litres of fluid intake in 24 hours. | Precise/concise statement of nursing actions.<br>1 Sit upright with use of back support and pillows.<br>2 2 hourly turns (10 a.m., 12 p.m., 2 p.m., 4 p.m., 6 p.m., 8 p.m., etc.).<br>3 180 ml of fluid at meal times and nourishing fluids and fruit juices in between meals. | | |

*Figure 7.3*   Problem-orientated care plan — teaching prompt, showing example of problems, outcome and care plan statements

| University of Manchester – Department of Nursing. M5/Assessment Unit | | |
|---|---|---|
| DAILY CARE PLAN FOR............................................................. | | |
| *Times* | *Daily Activities/Sleep and Rest* | *Progress* (Comments achieved or /X) |
| Awakening 8 a.m. | | |
| 9 a.m. | | |
| 10 a.m. | | |
| 11 a.m. | | |
| 12 noon | | |
| 1 p.m. | | |
| 2 p.m. | | |
| 3 p.m. | | |
| 4 p.m. | | |
| 5 p.m. | | |
| 6 p.m. | | |
| 7 p.m. | | |
| 8 p.m. | | |
| 9 p.m. | | |
| 10 p.m. | | |
| NIGHT TIME | | |
| | | |
| | | |
| | | |

**Figure 7.4**  Daily care plan

| University of Manchester – Department of Nursing. M5/Assessment Unit | | |
|---|---|---|
| DAILY CARE PLAN FOR............................................................. | | |
| _Times_ | _Daily Activities/Sleep and Rest_ | _Progress_ (Comments achieved or /X) |
| Awakening | Usually at 7 a.m. likes to use commode at bedside and then have a cup of tea | |
| 8 a.m. | Sit out in chair by bedside for breakfast. Add extra bran to diet | |
| 9 a.m. to | EITHER – 1. Encourage to wash hands and face at bedside, plus shave with electric razor | |
| 10 a.m. | OR – 2. Encourage up, bath and shave in bathroom. Help with dressing | |
| 11 a.m. | Take B.P. and pulse. Encourage fluids min. of 180 mls. Likes coffee – no milk no sugar | |
| 12 noon | Give medications prior to lunch at 12.15 p.m. Encourage patient to walk with special frame | |
| 1 p.m. | To dining-room, walk back to bedside and allow patient to either rest in chair or on his bed | |
| 2 p.m. to | For 1 hour – Take B.P. and pulse + temperature Check pulmonary function with Wright's peak flow meter | |
| 3 p.m. | Record result in notes | |
| 4 p.m. | Exercises as per chart in day room Encourage fluids min. of 180 mls. – likes tea, no sugar | |
| 5 p.m. | Walk to dining-room for evening meal | |
| 6 p.m. | Usually likes – sandwiches, fruit and tea | |
| 7 p.m. | Encourage to walk to day room, likes to watch T.V. or read evening paper | |
| 8 p.m. | Encourage to walk to day room, likes to watch T.V. or read evening paper | |
| 9 p.m. to | Walk back to bedside, likes to be in bed by 9.30 p.m. | |
| 10 p.m. | Take to toilet prior to this – likes a drop of whisky (30 mls.), no night sedation needed | |
| NIGHT TIME | | |
| 1 a.m. | Usually wakes to use commode at bedside – may only need to pass urine. Therefore encourage use of urinal | |
| 6 a.m. | Usually awake – but does not like to be disturbed until 7 a.m. | |
| | | |

**_Figure 7.5_**   Completed example of a daily care plan

Another reason for developing a daily care plan is preparation for transferring a patient home; if possible, try to encourage relatives, friends and the district nurse to be involved in this planning. For example:

| Time | Patient activity while in hospital | Proposed patient activity at home | Comments |
|------|-----------------------------------|-----------------------------------|----------|
|      |                                   |                                   |          |

## The standard care plan

The third type of care plan which may be helpful is the standard care plan (*Figures 8.1–8.7*). This is basically a checklist of the routine care which it is proposed to give a patient, irrespective of his specific needs. It should be arrived at by careful evaluation of what has been carried out in the past for patients with similar needs. All actions should be based on sound scientific principles and research findings. Periodically, it should be up-dated and revised; therefore a special standard care planning committee should be formed to carry this out every six months.

One criticism of this approach is that it goes against the philosophy of individualising care planning. However, this approach cuts down unnecessary written work and establishes safe and helpful routines of nursing care. It leaves more time to concentrate on plans for the specific and individual problems of the patient.

## 8

# Implementation in Practice

## Nursing actions

As stated in Part I, the stage of implementation involves putting the plan of care into action or carrying out the prescribed nursing care. Some examples of care plans are given in this text and from these it will be seen that nursing actions can be such as:

'Position slowly.'
'Assist when up as long as dizziness persists.'
'Sterile technique with dressing change.'
'Listen to and encourage expression of fears and concerns.'

This means there is a variety of nursing actions including physical and psychological help and support, counselling and teaching. The care plan format provides a space to record the date on which specific nursing actions are started and that on which they are discontinued. There is also a section for recording 'Progress'. While implementing the nursing care plan it is important that progress notes are written. They form the basis of evaluation, but it is only as the care is being carried out that some of the patient responses or 'Expected outcomes' can be observed.

## Organisation of nursing care

In wards where nursing work is allocated on a job assignment basis, lists of jobs are made and nurses are allocated tasks. Where the nursing process is used the prescription of nursing care and the nursing action is more usually carried out on a basis of patient assignment or team nursing. In this way, the implementation of the nursing care plan for any one patient can be co-ordinated and carried out by one or two nurses who assume responsibility for his care. This has the advantage of promoting consistency in the care of the patient, reducing the number of nurses to whom he has to relate, and bringing all the tasks for his care together so that they can be carried out with less frequent disturbance of the patient. In the professorial nursing unit at Manchester Royal Infirmary a modified system of 'primary nursing' has been developed; that is, the way in which work was organised to implement the nursing process and carry out prescribed nursing care was recognised as that called 'primary nursing' in the literature.

| NAME | | | Hospital No. | | |
|---|---|---|---|---|---|
| | | | | _Tick when completed_ | |
| | MASTER OR STANDARD PRE-OPERATIVE CARE PLAN | | | _Date/Time_ | |
| _Date Commenced_ | _Patient's Nursing Problem_ | _Expected Outcome_ | _Nursing Care Plan_ | _Discontinued_ | _Signature_ |
| When admitted. Prior to operation. | 1 Safe and reasonable pre-op. preparation.  To reduce pre- and post-operative physical/ psychological stress, wound infections, pain, inhalation of stomach contents, and to ensure that right patient receives correct operation. | 1 Completed pre-op. assessment and care plan with patient prepared for theatre and able to express any anxieties and difficulties. | 1(a) Obtain and record baseline vital signs (temp., pulse., resp., B.P. test urine, weight).<br>(b) Note and record any significant factors from past medical history (e.g. drug allergies, respiratory difficulties).<br>(c) Note and record any loose teeth or other problems that might affect post-op. management.<br>(d) Plan pre-op. teaching.<br>(e) Enquire and shave if desired operation site.<br>(f) Bath (remove make-up – don't use talc.).<br>(g) Check identity-band, completed consent form, notes, X-rays.<br>(h) Starve from ........ (no less than 4 hours).<br>(i) Remove prosthesis – dentures, hair-piece, contact lenses, rings<br>(j) Use of operation gown and disposable pants.<br>(k) Safe keeping – security of valuables.<br>(l) Emotional support by talking to patient and encouraging ventilation of fears, reassurance.<br>(m) Check and give pre-med.<br>(n) Empty bladder.<br>(o) Escort to theatre. | | |

_Figure 8.1_   Master or standard pre-operative care plan

| NAME | MASTER OR STANDARD POST-OPERATIVE CARE PLAN | | | Hospital No. | | |

| Date Commenced | Patient's Nursing Problem | Expected Outcome | Nursing Care Plan | Tick when completed | |
| | | | | Date/Time Discontinued | Signature |
|---|---|---|---|---|---|
| Immediately on return to ward. | 1 Potential lung congestion and blocked airway due to anaesthesia and inactivity. | 1(a) Normal breathing pattern.<br>(b) Temp. under 38°C.<br>(c) Clear lung sounds.<br>(d) No signs of cyanosis.<br>(24-hr. deadline) | 1(a) Semi-prone position.<br>(b) Guedel airway in situ until patient swallowing.<br>(c) Stay with pt. until regained consciousness.<br>(d) ½ hrly temp. – change when stable.<br>(e) Oxygen and suction near at hand.<br>(f) Encourage deep breathing and coughing, with help, when conscious. | | |
| | 2(a) Potential shock due to bleeding and/or anaesthesia.<br>(b) Hypovolaemia. | 2(a) Stable B.P.<br>(b) Pulse 60–100.<br>(c) No bright red bleeding.<br>(d) No blood saturated dressings.<br>(24-hr. deadline) | 2(a) ½ hrly observations of B.P., temp., pulse. (change to hourly – 2 hrly if stable.)<br>(b) Check dressings.<br>(c) Call doctor if shock occurs or bleeding – elevate. Apply more dressings on top. | | |
| | 3 Potential fluid and electrolyte imbalance due to anaesthetic, operative procedure and/or analgesics. | 3(a) Taking and retaining fluids.<br>(b) Electrolytes within normal limits. | 3(a) Check I.V. infusion regime.<br>(b) Oral hygiene.<br>(c) Ice chips to suck followed by clear liquids as pt. tolerates.<br>(d) Use of fluid balance chart.<br>(e) Record/report difficulties. | | |
| | 4 Pain in surgical area due to operative procedure. | 4(a) Verbal expression of reasonable comfort.<br>(b) Post-op. pain medication controls pain. | 4(a) Offer pain medication.<br>(b) Change pt.'s position frequently/2 hrly. | | |

*Figure 8.2*  Master or standard post-operative care plan

NAME                                    Hospital No

MASTER OR STANDARD POST-OPERATIVE CARE PLAN

| Date Commenced | Patient's Nursing Problem | Expected Outcome | Nursing Care Plan | Tick when completed Date/Time Discontinued | Signature |
|---|---|---|---|---|---|
| Within 24 hrs | 5 Potential urinary retention due to bladder atony from anaesthesia. | 5(a) Voiding within 8 hrs a total of 240 ml. (b) No bladder distension. (c) No pain in lower abdomen, or discomfort. | 5(a) Maintain and report urinary output. (b) Fluid balance chart. (c) Sit upright. Encourage to void. | | |
| | 6 Potential wound infection due to bacterial invasion. | 6(a) Clean dry wound. (b) Temp. below 38°C. (c) No redness or oedema of wound. | 6(a) Sterile technique with dressing change. (b) Inspect operative site for potential problems. (c) Don't allow dressings to soak through. | | |
| | 7 Potential ileus, gas pains and/or constipation due to anaesthetic or surgical trauma. | 7(a) Abdomen soft and flat. (b) Passing flatus. (c) Bowel movement by third day. | 7(a) Keep active in bed. (b) Use rectal/flatus tube PRN. (c) Use laxatives on medical advice. (d) Check bowel sounds. | | |
| | 8 Potential anxiety and stress due to unknown outcome of surgery and/or change in life-style and body image. | 8(a) Verbalises fears and concerns regarding outcome. | 8(a) Spend 15 mins. on average per shift with patient – listening and encouraging. (b) Discuss surgery. (c) Encourage early ambulation. | | |
| | 9 Potential problem of mobility complications following surgical intervention and/or anaesthetic. | 9(a) No signs/symptoms of deep vein thrombosis, or immobility. | 9(a) Encourage foot and leg exercises. (b) Discourage from crossing legs – do not use pillows under calves. (c) Mobilise patient and sit out of bed, following consultation with surgeon, as soon as possible. | | |

*Figure 8.2*   continued

NAME _____

STANDARD CARE PLAN: INTRAVENOUS PYELOGRAM

Hospital No. _____

| Date Commenced | Patient's Nursing Problem | Expected Outcome | Nursing Care Plan | Tick when completed Date/Time Discontinued | Signature |
|---|---|---|---|---|---|
| | 1 Potential problem of bladder and ureters being obscured from view by faeces and urine. | 1 Clear view of bladder and ureters. | 1 Empty bowel. (a) Clear fluids from evening before. (b) ½ bottle X prep. between 2 and 4 p.m. the day before. (c) Light breakfast on day of appointment. 2 Empty bladder prior to appointment. | | |
| | 2 Understanding of procedure. Reduction in anxiety, and expression of fears by patient. | 2 Understanding of procedure and reduction in anxiety with expression of fears by patient. | 1 Explain briefly about procedure and date when first known. 2 Day before explain in detail: (a) Prep. required. (b) The time of appointment. (c) The place. (d) Details of the actual procedure. (e) Length of time away from ward. (f) What will be wearing. (g) That meal or snack will be available on return to ward. | | |
| | 3 Clothing. | 3 Wear X-ray gown. | 1 Put on X-ray gown ½ hour before appointment. | | |

*Figure 8.3*   Standard care plan for an intravenous pyelogram

STANDARD CARE PLAN: BARIUM ENEMA

NAME _____   Hospital No. _____

| Date Commenced | Patient's Nursing Problem | Expected Outcome | Nursing Care Plan | Tick when completed Date/Time Discontinued | Signature |
|---|---|---|---|---|---|
| | 1 Faeces in lower bowel. | 1 Clear lower bowel to allow clear X-ray of rectum and colon. | 1 Fluids only from evening the day before.<br>2 Disposable enema before going to bed.<br>3 Rectal washout 1 hour before barium enema. | | |
| | 2 No knowledge of procedure – potential problem of anxiety. | 2 Clear understanding of procedure and reduction in anxiety with expression of fears by patient. | 1 2 days before explain briefly about procedure and in more detail preparation required.<br>2 Day before explain in detail:<br>(a) The time.<br>(b) The place.<br>(c) What will be wearing.<br>(d) Details of procedure.<br>(e) Length of time in X-ray.<br>(f) When next meal will be. | | |
| | 3 Clothing. | 3 To wear X-ray gown. | 1 Put on X-ray gown ½ hour before appointment. | | |
| | 4 Discomfort and soiling with barium following procedure. | 4 Clean and comfortable. | 1 Offer bath or wash.<br>2 Allow to dress in fresh clean clothes. | | |

*Figure 8.4*   Standard care plan for a barium enema

| NAME | | Hospital No. | | | |
|---|---|---|---|---|---|

STANDARD CARE PLAN: BARIUM MEAL / SWALLOW

| Date Commenced | Patient's Nursing Problem | Expected Outcome | Nursing Care Plan | Tick when completed | |
|---|---|---|---|---|---|
| | | | | Date/Time Discontinued | Signature |
| | 1 Food in stomach. | 1 Empty stomach to allow clear X-ray of oesophagus and stomach. | 1 Starve for 6 hours before appointment. | | |
| | 2 No knowledge of procedure – potential problem of anxiety. | 2 Clear understanding of procedure. Reduction in anxiety, and expression of fears by patient. | 2 Explain briefly procedure and date when first known. (a) Prep. required, i.e. no food or drink from........ (state time). (b) The time. (c) The place. (d) Length of time. (e) What will be wearing. (f) Detail of procedure. (g) That meal will be available on return to ward. | | |
| | 3 Clothing. | 3 To wear X-ray gown. | 1 Put on X-ray gown ½ hour before appointment. | | |
| | 4 Bad taste from barium in mouth following X-ray. | 4 Clean mouth and patient reports 'no foul taste'. | 1 Provide mouthwash on return to ward. 2 Provide drink of patient's choice. | | |

*Figure 8.5*  Standard care plan for a barium meal/swallow

STANDARD CARE PLAN: GASTROSCOPY

NAME

Hospital No.

| Date Commenced | Patient's Nursing Problem | Expected Outcome | Nursing Care Plan | Tick when completed Date/Time Discontinued | Signature |
|---|---|---|---|---|---|
| Pre-operative | 1 Potential problem of food in stomach. | Empty stomach. 1 Prevention of vomit and aspiration. 2 Clear view of stomach lining. | 1 Starve for 6 hours before appointment. 2 Premedication before appointment as prescribed. | | |
| | 2 No knowledge of procedure – potential problem of anxiety prior to procedure. | 1 Relaxed, patient who has a clear understanding and is able to express any anxieties. | 1 Explain briefly about procedure and date when first known. 2 Day before explain in detail: (a) Prep. required, i.e. no food and drink. (b) The time. (c) The place. (d) The actual procedure. (e) Length of time. (f) What will be wearing. (g) Unable to eat for 4 hours afterwards. | | |
| Post-operative | 3 Potential problem of spasm of oesophagus and aspiration of food content for 4 hours after procedure, due to effects of anaesthetic on throat and swallowing reflex. | 1 Empty stomach for 4 hours – prevention of reflux and aspiration. | 1 No food or drink for 4 hours after procedure. 2 Allow sips of water at first. 3 Then fluids. 4 Then soft foods. 5 Finally when all tolerated can take normal diet. | | |

*Figure 8.6*　Standard care plan for gastroscopy

### MASTER CARE PLAN: MYELOGRAM

DEFINITION:
Introduction of a dye into the subarachnoid space of the spinal canal for X-ray visualisation of a lesion, disc, or compression of cord.

DAY BEFORE X-RAY PREPARATION:
(1) Explain procedure and reason to be done to patient/family.
(2) Give and review booklet on *Myelogram* from Patient Education.
(3) Verify and document patient/family verbal understarding.
(4) Check that permit was obtained by physician.

MORNING OF X-RAY PREPARATION:
(1) Give clear liquid breakfast.
(2) Complete A.M. care.
(3) Take and record T, P, R, B.P., neuro check.
(4) Complete pre-op. checklist.
(5) Give and chart pre X-ray medication as ordered.
(6) Send to X-ray; prepare room for patient's return.

POST X-RAY CARE:
(1) Receive patient from X-ray, position comfortably and flat in bed for 12–24 hours. If patient is very drowsy, position on side.
(2) Take and record, T, P, R, B.P., neuro check every 15 minutes X 4, every 30 minutes X 2, every hour X 2, then every 4 hours for 24 hours or as ordered.
(3) Observe for signs of meningeal irritation – neck rigidity, Kernig's sign (passive extension of leg with thigh flexed is restricted and causes pain), photophobia, fever, irritability.
(4) Review physician's orders and call H.O. for any problems.
(5) Force p.o. fluids, serve diet as ordered, record I&O. Check each voiding for specific gravity until value is below 1.020.
(6) Give analgesics as ordered for headache.
(7) Check extremity strength and movement with vital signs.
(8) Document procedure, post X-ray care, patient response and toleration.

Prepared by:   Pat Aucoin, R.N.
Date:          April, 1978

The North Carolina Memorial Hospital
Department of Nursing

*Figure 8.7*   Master or standard care plan for myelogram — example from North Carolina

# Primary nursing

References on the subject of primary nursing are few in the UK nursing literature. Two recently notable exceptions are those of Kratz (1979) and Lee (1979).

Manthey, the initial innovator of primary nursing who developed this method of organising nursing care at the University of Minnesota hospitals, outlines its characteristics (Manthey *et al.*, 1970). Manthey's main aim was to develop a pattern of care that would permit nurses to take on more individual responsibility for fewer patients, and provide them with comprehensive care. This resulted in the formation of two kinds of personnel — 'primary nurses' and 'associate nurses'. A primary nurse is responsible for the care of patients throughout their stay in the hospital, and an associate nurse is someone who cares for a patient whose primary nurse is off duty. The primary nurse/patient ratio is in the region of 1 to 4 on day duty, depending upon the type of care needed and the rapidity of patient turn-over.

Primary nursing could be confused with the terms 'primary health care' and 'the primary care team' as used in the UK. This is the first level of care which a client receives in the health-care system either in a casualty department at a hospital or, more usually, by the primary care team of doctors, nurses and social workers in the community.

Ciske (1974), who worked as Consultant in Rehabilitation Nursing at the University of Minnesota, with Manthey, outlines the five basic concepts in the primary nursing system:

1. Assignment of each patient to a specific (primary) nurse who usually provides his care each day she is on duty until the patient's discharge or transfer.

2. Patient assessment by the primary nurse, who plans the care to be given when she is not on duty, when secondary or associate nurses care for her patients. Thus, 24-hour responsibility for care is actualised through the primary nurse's written directives on Kardex and other communication tools.

3. Patient involvement in the care provided and identification of his goals relating to how the medical condition affects his life-style.

4. Care giver to care giver communication — both in the nursing staff's daily reporting methods and between disciplines.

5. Discharge planning — including patient teaching, family involvement, and appropriate referrals.

As Kratz and Lee found, primary nursing is not just confined to the USA; it is also well under way at the Sir Charles Gairdner Hospital in Perth, Western Australia. The major advantage of using this system of care for Australian nurses was the patient contact — being responsible for a person's care from admission to discharge.

## Development of primary nursing at Manchester Royal Infirmary

The term 'primary nursing' is not yet widely accepted in the UK. We came to develop and organise our nursing care along the Minnesota pattern at Manchester more by accident than design. One of the major factors which moved us in this direction was the use of the nursing process. We found that if we were going to carry out the stages of the nursing process, then to maintain continuity and avoid fragmentation the nurse who admitted the patient and took his history needed to follow the patient throughout his hospitalisation. Due to staffing shortages and the enthusiasm of the learners coming to the ward, we did not at first restrict this role to the registered nurses.

The following pattern of care has now emerged:

1. Each patient on the ward is allocated to a registered nurse who is responsible for:

   (a) Assessing, planning and implementing the nursing care and regularly up-dating the care plan.
   (b) Working with the patient every time she is on duty.
   (c) Following the patient's progress through hospitalisation.
   (d) Making home visits, sometimes prior, during and after discharge home.
   (e) Arranging transfer home.
   (f) Functioning as the patient's advocate.
   (g) Serving as the main co-ordinator of his total care.
   (h) Presenting his case at nursing care evaluation sessions.

2. Each patient on the ward is allocated to a second nurse (*Figure 8.8*), who is usually a learner or auxiliary, and who works very closely with the registered nurse and may take over some of the aspects of the nursing care. She will also be allocated to the patient, especially when the registered nurse is off duty.

3. It is not always possible to have primary and secondary nurses working opposite shifts to each other; therefore, all nurses on the ward serve as associates.

4. Where possible, primary nurses make themselves available for ward rounds and case discussions related to their patients.

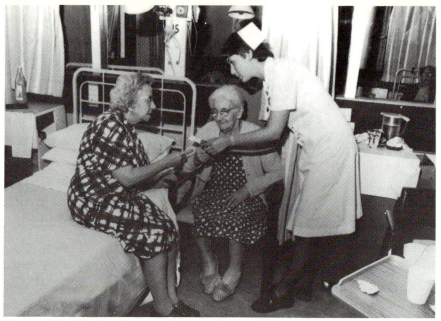

*Figure 8.8*   'Each patient on the ward is allocated to a second nurse.' Here, the second nurse is seen involved in patient teaching

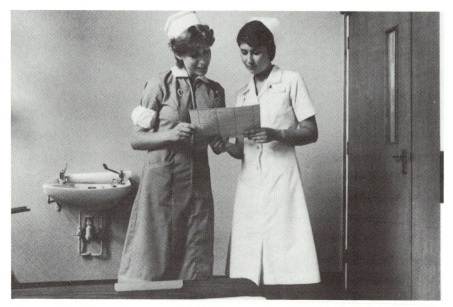

*Figure 8.9*   'The primary nurse discusses and questions carefully any major changes in the patient's nursing care plan, following off duty or days off.' Here, the primary nurse is seen discussing a care plan with a second nurse

5. The primary nurse discusses and questions carefully any major changes in the patient's nursing care plan, following periods off duty or days off (*Figure 8.9*).

6. One nurse will act as ward co-ordinator each day. Even though the sister is on duty, she may not assume this role.

7. The ward sister/charge nurse role fundamentally changes under this system; she is now able to:

   (a) Work on the ward more with patients and with nursing staff.

   (b) Take on the duties of a primary nurse, where her expertise is especially required.

   (c) Assign nurses to patients according to the care needs of patients and the abilities and/or case load of the staff nurses.

   (d) Continue to manage the ward, the patient environment, and facilitate the development of the holistic patient care approach, and the development of nursing staff.

There is no doubt that the key to success using primary nursing lies in the attitude of nursing staff. As Kratz (1979) reported from Australia, before this system spreads ward sisters have to be highly motivated and have the support of their colleagues and co-operation of medical staff.

Our medical staff at first found it a little strange that, instead of consulting the ward sister about each patient, they had to relate more to the rest of the trained nursing staff. The consultant on our ward certainly likes the greater depth of knowledge that the primary nurses have about their patients. In some hospitals the primary nurse's name is placed over each patient's bed. We have a large 'rub off' board showing the names, placed in the entrance to the ward. This not only helps the doctors but other health professionals, visitors, relatives and friends. The patient assignment sheet is given in *Figure 8.10*.

## Termination of relationships

A system of primary nursing or patient allocation promotes a far closer relationship between one patient and one nurse. This is more demanding and the nurse needs to plan for the termination of the relationship. Ending of the therapeutic nurse–patient relationship can evoke a wide variety of emotions. It is important, therefore, for the nurse to be alert to her own feelings as well as those of the patient.

Perhaps the most rewarding aspect of nursing a patient, using the nursing process, is that the nurse feels a sense of involvement and personal achievement. She has been responsible or directly involved in helping the patient recover, or in achieving a peaceful death. 'Happy staff who feel

| DAILY PATIENT ASSIGNMENT | | | | |
|---|---|---|---|---|
| Date | Team Members: Morning Shift | Patients | Team Members: Afternoon/ Evening/ Shift | Notes |
| | | | | |

**Figure 8.10**   Patient assignment sheet

respected by themselves and others not only gain more themselves but give more to their patients. The use of the nursing process makes it easier for the contribution of individual nurses to be recognised' (Ashworth and Castledine, 1980).

The patient or his relatives may have grown dependent on the physical and pyschological support of the nurse, and be fearful of that support being withdrawn. They may wish to give the nurse a gift. There are times when the expression of thanks or offering of a gift is not the end of the relationship, and the patient wishes it to continue. The nurse may have derived satisfaction from the 'giving' involved in nursing and may also wish to continue the relationship.

## When to start terminating the relationship

The stage of termination is set during the first interview with the patient when the nurse is introducing herself, describing the style of nursing care which is going to be carried out and her involvement; for instance, 'You will be with us for approximately three days, which means that I will be on duty and looking after you for most of that period'.

Following on from this conversation and the gathering of information, the nurse with the help of the patient clarifies the nursing care objectives or expected outcomes. It is these objectives or outcomes which will influence and help to determine the timing of termination; for instance, 'The purpose of your coming to this ward is to have the following tests; this means from a nursing point of view that our aim is to achieve the following . . . '.

This type of statement by the nurse helps to clarify her position in the overall treatment plan and care which the patient will be receiving.

## Recognising the feelings

Whatever feelings may be evoked by ending a relationship with a patient, there is no doubt that past experiences will be revived and brought into consideration. Edinburg, Zinberg and Kelman (1975) list these as:

(a) anger;

(b) rejection;

(c) abandonment;

(d) sadness;

(e) guilt;

(f) relief;

(g) pleasure;

(h) sense of independence;

(i) sense of accomplishment.

If a nurse has worked very closely for a long time with a patient, she may find it more difficult to terminate the relationship. For example, a nurse working in an intensive care unit may continually feel an obligation to visit her patient when he has been transferred to another ward. This situation may disrupt rather than help in the continuity of nursing care, as both the patient and the new ward nurses will be unsure of their involvement and goals. Too often nurses want to 'cling on' to the patients they like or have done a lot for. On the other hand, a nurse may start to reject or try to terminate a relationship too soon if she finds a particular patient difficult to care for.

Discussion with more experienced nursing colleagues is essential if we are to help nurses recognise their feelings and come to terms and deal with their own conflicts.

Patients themselves may become defensive and deny that termination is a significant experience or that they have feelings associated with it. This may lead to resistance and difficulties in transferring the patient home. For instance, the patient may complain that his symptoms are recurring or that new ones are developing.

If the nurse recognises this regressive behaviour in a patient she may need to review whether her behaviour is reinforcing the patient's need for her. The use of the patient's care plan, especially the review of the objectives of nursing care, can help in dealing with this situation.

## Summary

In the majority of cases, termination poses no problems for the nurse; however, it is important for her to recognise that difficulties may occur, particularly with the more intensive involvement in the nursing process, and that transfer of a patient is not always as smooth as one would wish. Terminations following any length of interaction can be an emotionally difficult and trying event. It is important, therefore, that the nurse prepares for it from the first interaction with the patient.

# Interruptions in primary nursing

## Drug rounds

There are many difficulties when carrying out primary nursing and these may lead to interruptions of this method of care. An example is the administration of patients' drugs. Several methods of how this can be achieved with the minimum of disruption are given below:

*Method 1.* This method involves the ward co-ordinator (if she is trained) making a drug round with the assistance of one nurse from each of the nurse-patient allocated groups. Each nurse only joins the round for her specific allocated patients.

*Method 2.* If there are enough trained members of staff and students in each allocated patient group, then two nurses (one trained and one untrained) will administer their own patients' drugs on consultation with other group leaders.

*Method 3.* In some cases, patients may themselves have the responsibility for taking their drugs. These may be kept in a locked portion of the bedside locker or in a special self-dispensing trolley. It would be the role of the nurse who was allocated to that particular patient to check whether the patient had taken his tablets. This method of patient responsibility for drug-taking is not widely used, but has the advantage of assessing how compliant the patient will be with regard to taking his medications on transfer from the ward.

*Method 4.* Many hospitals state that drug administration should be carried out by a trained member of staff with the assistance of a pupil or student nurse. There may be some instances where, because of safety and shortage of staff, the drug round becomes one of the few designated tasks on the ward.

# The multidisciplinary team and the nursing process

Multidisciplinary team care has been developing over the past few years, so that many different people may now be involved in caring for a patient.

It is important that the nurse monitors the effect of paramedical invo.vement and encourages such personnel (physiotherapists, occupational therapists, etc.) to communicate their findings and share their ideas (*Figure 8.11*).

It may be possible to develop multidisciplinary problem-orientated records, but there are some points to be taken into consideration first.

Sharing personal information about a patient with others must be carefully monitored. The patient must be told if such a multidisciplinary approach is being used on the ward.

Where many members of a multidisciplinary team are involved in the patient's care, it is important to ensure that the patient is not 'over-assessed' and put through repeated and unnecessary activities for the sake of professional status.

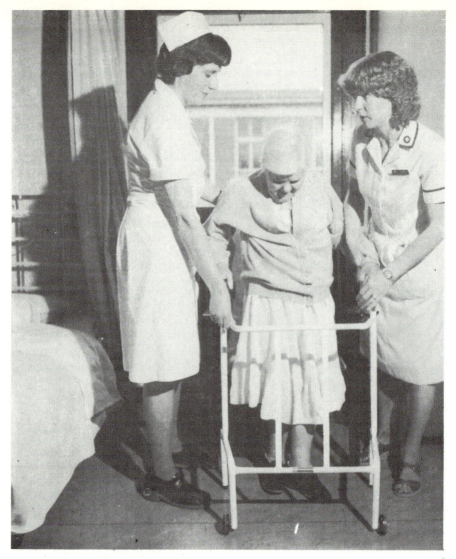

***Figure 8.11***   'It is important that the nurse monitors the effect of paramedical involvement and encourages such personnel (physiotherapists, occupational therapists, etc.) to communicate their findings and share their ideas'

## Transfer

Transferring a patient from hospital is often referred to as 'discharge'. We believe that this is an unfortunate term which tends to suggest that the nurse in hospital has completed all the nursing care required. There are many cases where such a belief is far from the truth, especially when what we have done is to shift the patient's nursing responsibility to another nursing agency.

Two methods of achieving successful transfer of a patient are given below:

1. The transfer of a photocopy of the patient's nursing records, plus a preliminary chat with district nurse colleagues or liaison nurse.

2. The completion of a nursing transfer summary form which includes a summary of the patient's nursing history and actual and potential problems. This, coupled with direct contact with the district nurse or liaison officer, can prove most valuable. *Figures 8.12(a)* and *8.12(b)* show a nursing transfer summary form, plus a sheet for problems and on-going nursing help, and *Figures 8.13(a)* and *8.13(b)* show a completed example of the forms.

## NURSING TRANSFER SUMMARY

Name of patient                                      Transfer date

Date of birth (age)                                  Method of transport

Patient's address                                    Home address
following transfer                                   (if different from opposite)


Next of kin or significant                           Length of stay
person to contact in emergency                       in hospital



Clinic visits scheduled


Patient's family/friends involved in post-transfer care




Referrals/community resources (including dates
contacted and by whom)




Medications



G.P. (name & address)

Profile/summary of patient

*Figure 8.12(a)*    Nursing transfer summary format

PATIENT'S PROBLEMS ON TRANSFER AND ON-GOING NURSING HELP

| Patient's Problems | Help being Given | Expected Outcome |
|---|---|---|
| | | |

Potential Risks

Contact nurse responsible ........................................... Date ......................
(Signature)
Address................................................................................
................................................................................

*Figure 8.12(b)*    Sheet for patient problems, help and outcome — this is the second part of the form in *Figure 8.12(a)*

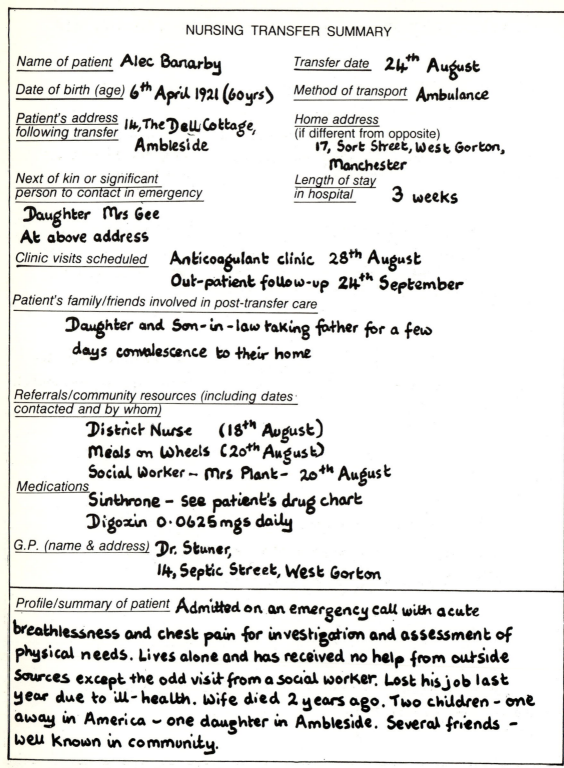

NURSING TRANSFER SUMMARY

*Name of patient* Alec Banarby

*Transfer date* 24th August

*Date of birth (age)* 6th April 1921 (60yrs)

*Method of transport* Ambulance

*Patient's address following transfer* 14, The Dell Cottage, Ambleside

*Home address (if different from opposite)* 17, Sort Street, West Gorton, Manchester

*Next of kin or significant person to contact in emergency*
Daughter Mrs Gee
At above address

*Length of stay in hospital* 3 weeks

*Clinic visits scheduled* Anticoagulant clinic 28th August
Out-patient follow-up 24th September

*Patient's family/friends involved in post-transfer care*
Daughter and Son-in-law taking father for a few days convalescence to their home

*Referrals/community resources (including dates contacted and by whom)*
District Nurse    (18th August)
Meals on Wheels (20th August)
Social Worker — Mrs Plank — 20th August

*Medications*
Sinthrone — see patient's drug chart
Digoxin 0.0625 mgs daily

*G.P. (name & address)* Dr. Stuner,
14, Septic Street, West Gorton

*Profile/summary of patient* Admitted on an emergency call with acute breathlessness and chest pain for investigation and assessment of physical needs. Lives alone and has received no help from outside sources except the odd visit from a social worker. Lost his job last year due to ill-health. Wife died 2 years ago. Two children - one away in America - one daughter in Ambleside. Several friends - well known in community.

**Figure 8.13(a)**   Completed example of a nursing transfer summary

PATIENT'S PROBLEMS ON TRANSFER AND ON-GOING NURSING HELP

| Patient's Problems | Help being Given | Expected Outcome |
|---|---|---|
| ① Potential problem of bleeding due to anticoagulant therapy | ① Teaching regarding signs and symptoms of bleeding and who to report to. | ① Patient able to verbalise the signs and symptoms of bleeding and knowledge of physical condition |
| ② Limited mobility due to poor heart condition. Difficulty walking long distances of 50-100 yards and getting up and down stairs. | ② Physiotherapy advice regarding climbing stairs and importance of rest when taking long walks. | ② Able to get out to shops and pub. Climb stairs 2 times daily. |
| ③ Small 1" x 1½" pressure sore on sacrum dry and healing - no signs of infection. | ③ Dry dressing daily. | ③ Healed area of skin and tissue by two weeks. |

Potential Risks

① "Blackouts" ? cerebral ischaemia ? hypotension

② Depression due to state of health and loneliness

③ Maintenance of an adequate diet

Contact nurse responsible ...J. Small...................... Date .24/8/81......
(Signature)
Address...... The General Hospital....................
.................. Ward 4.....................................

*Figure 8.13(b)*    Completed example of a sheet for patient problems, help and outcome — this is the second part of the form in *Figure 8.13(a)*

# 9

# Evaluation in Practice

One of the traditional methods of evaluating the outcomes of nursing care is to carefully examine the nursing notes or Kardex. In many cases, as Lelean (1973) has found, these nursing records are inadequate and usually consist of a series of insufficiently informative statements about what was done for the patient or comments expressing value judgements and conclusions without data to support the nurse's opinions, e.g. 'comfortable', 'better day', 'good night'.

Lelean found that 'written instructions in the Kardex report seldom augmented the verbal instructions and in some instances could contradict them'. When writing dependency statements about the patients on their wards, it has been also noted that many ward sisters are not fully aware of the condition of their patients. Many ward sisters still believe that it is the duty of the person in charge of the ward to write the progress notes on all the patients.

## Evaluation by objectives or expected outcomes

In Chapter 7 it was emphasised that the expected outcomes could be used as a basis for evaluation. The extent to which the patient's goals have been reached is used rather than on how well the nurse performs. We stated that 'the "expected outcome" is a statement of what the nurse expects the patient will be able to achieve by a certain time or date; that is, it is a statement of expected patient behaviour'.

Thus, using the nursing process system of collecting information and working with individual patients, demands that the information necessary for evaluating progress in the management of nursing problems is recorded in the progress notes. The recording of this information should, of course, be the responsibility of the nurse who has been assigned to look after the patient for a particular shift of duty.

Nursing care cannot be evaluated on the basis of brief comments which have no reference to the patient's nursing care plan.

One method of encouraging nurses to write progress notes in the nursing care plans is to write the number of the patient problem down and then comment about the progress which has been made. This can then be compared with the 'expected outcome'.

Weed (1970) states that progress notes are the most crucial part of the patient's record because 'they are the mechanism of follow-up on each problem'.

It is important therefore to write progress notes, as they not only indicate the current status and progress of the patient, but provide a valuable feedback of information which assists the nurse in redefining or up-dating the care plan if the desired outcomes have not been achieved.

As when taking the nursing history, information about the patient will not only come from the nurse's observations, but from:

(a) Statements and comments made by the patient, his family and friends.

(b) Comments and reports from other members of the health-care team.

(c) Laboratory reports, X-rays and reports from special procedures.

(d) Comments made at report and hand-over sessions including case conferences and ward rounds.

The nurse must be tuned in to this wide range of information and utilise sources of information as best she can in order to write a systematic and reliable report of the patient's progress. Lelean (1973) points out the importance and value of the nurse's records and stresses how in nursing situations the report is a legal document.

## Short-term or on-going evaluation

Not only will well written and clearly expressed progress notes form a good communication tool and legal record of nursing care, but they are an invaluable source of daily or on-going evaluation.

When writing the patient's progress notes, the nurse who has been giving the care should write up her observations. In some instances where an auxiliary nurse has carried out the nursing care based on the care plan, she should write the progress notes. (Auxiliary nurses will need help and instruction on how to do this and what they have written should be checked carefully by a trained nurse.)

Always refer to the patient's care plan when writing your notes (*Figure 9.1*). As stated earlier, one helpful method we have found is numbering the problems on the care plan, so that when the progress notes are written you write the number of the problem first and any significant observation or event relating to that problem after. Example:

(3) Patient walked about five feet today, with the aid of his walking frame; he still needs one nurse to supervise him.

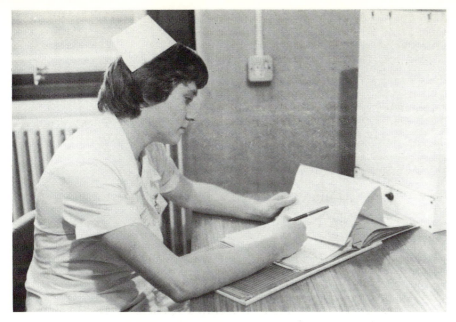

***Figure 9.1*** 'Always refer to the patient's care plan when writing your notes'

If there is no change in the care plan and nothing significant has happened during the shift when you have been caring for the patient, then you may record 'no change in care plan'.

It may be helpful, however, to record quotes from the patient on how he thinks and feels he is progressing. Example:

(3)  Patient states: 'I don't feel I am making any progress with my walking.'

When problems are resolved or a significant variation has taken place, then the problem on the care plan should be dated and discontinued.

If a problem recurs it does not receive its original number, but follows on in the sequence.

On occasions it may be necessary to rewrite a care plan because of the numerous crossings off and discontinuations. *Figures A.3, 9.2* and *9.6* show examples of progress notes.

# Points to consider when writing care plans and progress reports

1. Always write in ink.

2. Writing must be legible (if it is not, practise penmanship).

3. Use words that will be understood by everyone.

4. Be careful when using abbreviations; they may not be understood, and an over-abundance of them decreases communication.

5. The patient's name should be clearly stated on every sheet.

6. Always record the date and time of entrances.

7. Record carefully all events which have happened to the patient — even how he has tolerated sitting up in a chair may be significant.

8. Never erase notes; if an error is made, score a line through the mistake and write 'error' over the top. This may seem cumbersome but it prevents an accusation of having tampered with the record.

9. The nurse who made the observations or performed the procedure or carried out the care plan should chart the relevant information. If an auxiliary nurse is deemed capable of giving an aspect of the nursing care (plan) then she should chart or write about what she has done and its effect on the patient.

10. Full signatures should be used when signing notes.

11. It is important always to write observations and not conclusions of the patient's progress. Beware of recording speculations; it is the behaviour and events that lead up to these conclusions which should be recorded. Record what you *observed* and not what you think happened. Perhaps a good rule is the one which asks you to look at what you have written down and ask yourself the question: did you actually see what is written? Hear it? Smell it? Touch or taste it? If your answer to all these questions is 'No', then you have written a conclusion and not an observation.

12. Finally, do not forget to number the problems you are reviewing in your progress notes, so that an accurate evaluation can be made with regard to the problem to which you are referring.

PATIENT PROGRESS NOTES

| Date Ordered | Para-Nursing Involvement and Medical/Investigations | Date Completed | Progress/Evaluation |
|---|---|---|---|
| | This column is for use of paramedical staff and for noting any special medical tests and investigations. *For example:* M.S.S.U. (mid-stream specimen of urine) CXR (Chest X-Ray) Barium meal 24-hour urine collection Special blood tests Physiotherapy – special exercises Occupational therapy Dietician Chiropody | | Daily account (dated and signed) of patient's progress regarding nursing problems, objectives and plan of nursing care. Number comments and observations according to the patient's problems. Add significant comments made by the patient. |

*Figure 9.2*  Patient progress notes — teaching prompt

| Costello | David Patrick |
|---|---|
| Surname | Forename(s) |

**Address:** 38 Hatt Court, Rusholme, Manchester 20

| Next of Kin: Step-son Nathan Black, partially sighted and diabetic, history of depression (S/A)<br><br>Sister: visits him but has recently suffered a stroke | Date of Birth: 2 - 12 - 98<br>Age: 82 years |
|---|---|
| Likes to be referred to as: David | Relevant Tel. Nos.<br><br>Step-son Nathan Black (S/A)<br>225 - 4086 |

| Date of Admission to Hospital: 15 - 7 - 81 | Ward: M5 GAW |
|---|---|

**General Practitioner:** Dr. R. N. Tomlinson   Tel: 222 - 522618

**Reason for Admission:**
To give relative a rest

**Medical Diagnosis:** Cancer of the Prostate with spinal secondaries LVF and Ischaemic Heart Disease

**Consultant:** Dr. Brown

**What Patient or Family understands about his/her condition:**

Patient does not know he has cancer; he believes that the cause of his pain is arthritis. Step-son knows that he has cancer; he thinks that his step-father will go to pieces if he finds out that he has cancer.

**Patient's and/or Family Reaction to Hospital Admission:**

Mr. Costello is not worried as he is pleased to give his step-son a rest.

**Home Conditions:** Lives in OAP council flat since 1972 on 7th floor (lift). Bathroom and two bedrooms heated by electric fires. Lives with step-son who cares for him. No apparent difficulties on discharge.

*Figure 9.3*   Completed example of nursing progress notes (first stage nursing history)

| History taken from | |
|---|---|
| Mr. D. P. Costello | |
| | Record No.   431141 |

**Meaningful Person in Life:**                   Significant others/pets:

Step-son Nathan Black, age 62 years, partially sighted, diabetic and depressive history (lived with him for 38 years). Has sister who lives near (recent CVA).

**Community Resources (D.N.H.V., Social Worker, Meals on Wheels etc. . . .):**

Visited by Mr. Tatt (district nurse) daily to help with hygiene needs.

No meals on wheels or home help (doesn't like to have one).

**General Health History & Previous Hospital Admission:**   (1955) laparotomy and appendicectomy. (1966) partial gastrectomy. (1975) myocardial infarction and LVF. (1975) Ca prostate with spinal secondaries. (1980) Excision of rodent ulcer on forehead and papilloma on thigh.
1980 — MS to give son a rest (August)

**Religious Practices or Beliefs Patient finds helpful:**   Roman Catholic priest visits once a month to give Communion helpful and important to him.

**Recreational Activities and Past/Present Work Life:**   Likes watching TV and reading. Owned antique shop. Was a plasterer. Worked till 75 years old.

**General Assessment on Admission:**   B.P. $\frac{130}{70}$   P = 58   R = 20   T = 37°C   Knoll Scale = 14. Mobile with stick (has fallen recently). Moves all limbs. Has had problems sleeping in past — controlled now with sedatives. Likes to rest during day. Poor appetite — mainly liquids, soups, porridge. No nausea or vomiting. Has a tendency to constipation; continent — but occasionally "dribbles". Urine test = NAD pH 6 colour amber. Drinks fluids o.k. — tea, water, orange not coffee. No dehydration or oedema. False teeth not worn. Dyspnoea on exertion. History of angina. Pillows = 4. Peripheral circulation - o.k. Weight 52.9 kg. Feels excessive pain in stomach and back only relieved by analgesia. Speech, hearing and sight o.k. Skin condition o.k. Not able to dress/wash himself without aid. Very pleasant man, orientated, good conversational ability. Tendency to be quiet and withdrawn?

*N.B.*   Note the name of the person who carried out the assessment and if patient or relative or both  involved

| Signature   S. A. Kirkham | Date   15/7/81 |
|---|---|

*Figure 9.3*   continued

**David Costello**    CARE PLAN    431141

| Date Commenced | Patient's Nursing Problem | Expected Outcome | Nursing Care Plan | Tick when completed | |
|---|---|---|---|---|---|
| | | | | Date/Time Discontinued | Signature |
| 17/7/81 | 1) Patient is dyspnoeic (especially on exertion), due to angina. | 1) Patient will become less breathless (by activities controlled to patient's condition). | 1) (a) Pace nursing actions to patient abilities – time over washing, dressing, rests when mobilising. (b) Relieve any anxiety. Maintain calm atmosphere. (c) Prop up patient when in bed or in chair. (d) Encourage deep breathing and expectoration. | | |
| | 2) Patient has severe pain in abdomen and spine, due to medical condition. | 2) Pain is kept under control, and patient expresses satisfaction regarding this. | 2) (a) Ensure analgesia is given as required. (b) Distract patient e.g. reading. (c) Keep patient comfortable according to patient's wishes. | | |
| | 3) Patient is unable to see to his own hygiene needs, due to poor physical condition. | 3) Maintain hygiene and decrease dependence, and patient expresses satisfaction regarding this. | 3) (a) Help with wash or bath. (b) Observe mouth/eye condition. (c) Encourage patient to do as much as he can re: washing/dressing. | | |
| | 4) Patient often has dribbling of urine, due to medical condition. | 4) Keep patient continent, and patient expresses satisfaction regarding measures used to control incontinence. | 4) (a) Offer bottle regularly or encourage patient to use toilet. (b) If persists chart incontinence to establish pattern. (c) Keep patient clean and dry. | | |

*Figure 9.4*  Completed example of nursing progress notes (the nursing problem-orientated care plan)

CARE PLAN

| Date Commenced | Patient's Nursing Problem | Expected Outcome | Nursing Care Plan | Tick when completed Date/Time Discontinued | Signature |
|---|---|---|---|---|---|
| | 5) Has low nutritional status. Weight = 52.9 kgs. | 5) Improvement in nutrition. Maintain weight at 56 - 58 kgs. | 5)(a) Encourage patient to eat as much of meals as he can. (b) Supplement with Complan/Build-up. (c) Does patient need prescribed supplement? Discuss with medical staff and dietician. | | |
| | 6) Has tendency towards constipation. | 6) Bowels opened every day or as patient requires (usual daily pattern). | 6)(a) Add bran to soup and porridge. (b) Encourage mobilisation. (c) Administer laxative if required. | | |
| | 7) Liable to develop pressure sores. | 7) Pressure sores prevented. | 7)(a) Ensure sheepskin is in bed. (b) Turn 2 - 4 hourly in bed and walk when sitting in chair. (c) Observe areas - heels, sacrum etc. (d) Keep clean and dry and improve nutritional status. | | |
| | 8) History of sleeping problems. | 8) Sleeps for 8 - 9 hours (patient's normal pattern). | 8)(a) Administer prescribed sedative. (b) Discuss any problems, worries. (c) Make patient comfortable. | | |

*Figure 9.4* continued

**IN-DEPTH ASSESSMENT**

Date...16/7/81......    Name....David...Costello..........    Hospital No....43114 1

Nurse....Kirkham...

*Activity and Movement*  Uses walking stick to walk with. Can walk moderate distances without aid, becomes breathless so needs to rest when mobilising. Moves all limbs. Can move from chair to bed unaided. Moves himself when in bed. Needs help with washing and dressing.

*Rest and Sleep*  History of problems with sleeping, always requires sedation. N.B. Patient states that Nitrazepam is ineffective. Likes to go to bed about 9.30p.m. and then sleeps through until 6.30 a.m. Prefers to have a rest after lunch. Does not like bed rails.

*Nutrition*  Poor appetite. Mainly eats soft/fluid diet - especially soup, fish and ice cream, porridge. Generally eats at every meal time. N.B. Patient has had a partial gastrectomy. No nausea/vomiting. Indigestion when eats too much. Weight 52·9 kgs. Appears slightly undernourished.(Possible lack of vitamin C and protein). No apparent anaemia.

*Elimination/Continent State*  Tendency to constipation. Takes aperient at home each night and bran in his porridge on morning at home. States that he has not opened bowels for 3 days. His normal "routine" = daily. No problems of pain passing urine through occasionally incontinent - "dribbling" - urine test - NAD ph 5, colour amber, uses and asks for bottle satisfactorily.

*Fluids and Electrolytes*  Drinks satisfactory amount - with and between meals. Likes orange and tea, dislikes coffee. No signs of dehydration/oedema. Has false teeth but prefers not to wear them because it makes his mouth sore.

*Oxygenation and Circulation*  Is dyspnoeic on exertion. No cyanosis or clubbing of fingers. Needs at least 4 pillows when in bed. Sometimes has pain in his chest. Suffers from angina on effort. Peripheral circulation appears to be satisfactory but veins of hand are prominent.

*Regulation and Senses*

B.P. 130/70, P. = 58, R. = 20, T. = 37°C.  Wears glasses for reading. Hearing, smell, temperature of skin - normal.

*Figure 9.5*    Completed example of a more in-depth assessment (replacing second level assessment, shown previously, and following a systems approach)

IN-DEPTH ASSESSMENT

Date..16/7/81....            Name.....David. Costello....            Hospital No.....4.3.1141...    Nurse...Kirkham............

Skin Condition    No wounds, ulcers or pressure areas. Hair and nail condition satisfactory.

Emotional State

Perception of Health    Accepts being ill as "one of those things". Sees no future only death, which he is not frightened about he says.

Conversational Ability    Alert, orientated to time, person and place. Good long term and short term memory. Good conversational ability.

Significant Non-Verbal Gestures    Sits quietly thinking.

Usual Reactions to Stressful Events    Feels that he copes well with problems in life. Tries to reason out problems to himself.

Observable Behaviour and Mood Swings    Anxious only over the trouble he causes others. Sometimes he becomes depressed but only temporarily. Generally tries to stay calm. May be withdrawn but only because he is quiet. Pleasant gentleman who seems fairly happy.

Figure 9.5    continued

PART OF PATIENT'S PROGRESS NOTES

Date................

Name...David Costello....................

Hospital No....43.1141....

**Day Report – S.A.Kirkham**

19/7/81

1) Dyspnoea only when moving from chair to bed or walking.
2) Analgesia required (Panadeine Co and Naprlen both given twice today). Patient stated that he felt "a lot better today than I have been feeling."
3) Able to wash himself using bowl by bed, needing help only with dressing.
4) Using toilet and commode as required. No incontinence.
5) Had no breakfast, but had soup and sweet for lunch.
6) No complaints.
7) Skin condition stable, patient moves about as he wishes. Patient goes to table for meals and seems to enjoy contact with other patients.

S.A.Kirkham

**Night Report – T.May**

20/7/81

1) No signs of breathing difficulties during the night, slept with 3 pillows.
2) No medication given since 9 p.m. States that his pain "much better now tablets have been changed."
3) As plan
4) Continent during the night.
5) Extra feeds as charted.
6) Bowels not opened during night.
7) No signs of soreness.
8) Says he has slept well – sedation given at 9 p.m. with analgesic.

T.May

*Figure 9.6*   Example of part of progress notes

# Patient-centred ward conferences

Another method of evaluating the patient's progress, and in particular the nursing contribution, is to hold a patient care conference.

Such a conference could be attended by nurses only (with inputs from nursing management and education), or they could include medical and paramedical staff or the patient and his family and friends (*Figure 9.7*). Whoever attends, the main reasons for holding a conference are as follows:

1. To focus on 'expected outcomes' which have not been fully achieved.

2. To make time for reviewing assessment, problem identification and the nursing care which has been given.

3. To help plan for the transfer of the patient to another hospital or home.

4. For nurses to develop new and wider understandings of their patients.

5. To review the research findings and see if any are applicable to the patient's nursing care.

6. To give members of the nursing team the opportunity to develop managerial and inter-personal communication skills.

Timings of the conferences should coincide with the various periods of the patient's progress on the ward, and usually the nurse who has been most concerned with the patient (the primary nurse) will present her case to those attending.

There is a danger sometimes that helpful comments may be seen as major criticisms and lapses in nursing care; it is therefore important to support the case presenter by a positive atmosphere. The conference should be built around the following areas:

1. Orientation of the group to the patient and his family and friends. This should include all aspects of the patient's physical and psychosocial background.

2. The nursing and general health problems of the patient. Sometimes it is helpful to have the doctor presenting the medical facts and the nurse the nursing facts. In this way the nursing care activities implicated by the medical plan can be discussed.

3. The patient and his family's adjustment to the health problem.

4. The rationale for the prescription of nursing care and its implications for the assessment of problems and nursing action.

5. The identification of further possible problems and plans for nursing action.

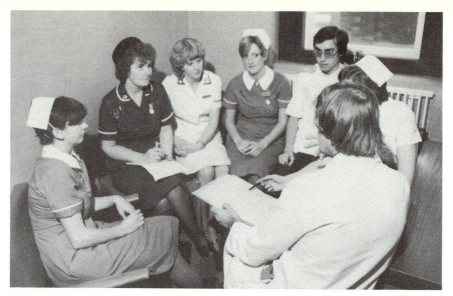

*Figure 9.7*   A patient-centred ward conference 'could include medical and paramedical staff.' Here, the conference has a physiotherapist and a district nurse in attendance

It is important that such conferences should be group-centred, and not leader-centred with the charge nurse or ward sister dominating what goes on. The leader, however, does not necessarily have to be the person in charge of the ward, so long as the appointed person:

(a)  Arranges the time and place of the conference well in advance.

(b)  Informs everybody of what is happening.

(c)  Arranges the chairs so that all the members can see and hear without difficulty.

(d)  Organises all the patients' relevant notes and any support papers and research reports.

(e)  Keeps to time and chairs the sesssion.

There is no doubt that arranging and conducting care conferences requires a special technique. The most important thing is to 'start small', by keeping the numbers down and keeping to a strict time limit.

When conducting a conference it is important to establish a happy, relaxed and non-threatening atmosphere. Continuous attention should be given to the nursing aspects of the case and the contribution by all the staff. Attention to factors which create a favourable work environment should be attended to carefully and problems in inter-personal relationships avoided.

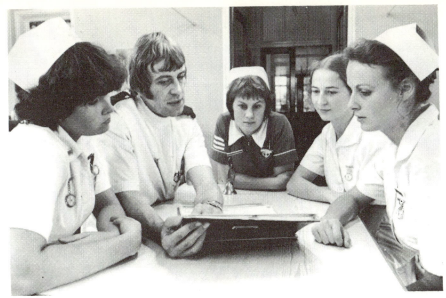

***Figure 9.8***    Daily report sessions: 'If the nursing process is being used, the nurse should review systematically the stated patient's problems and nursing orders on the care plan'

When drawing such a conference to a close, it is important that the chairman summarises what has been said and outlines further areas of nursing action.

## Daily report sessions

Patient care conferences should not replace daily report sessions, at which each member of the team who has been looking after a particular patient has the opportunity to present the patient's progress to the rest of the staff. In the past, Lelean (1973) has found that such report sessions have been a one-way process, usually from sisters to nurses. If the nursing process is being used, the nurse should review systematically the stated patient's problems and nursing orders on the care plan (*Figure 9.8*) and then leave a few minutes for general discussion of observations and progress. It is important for the ward co-ordinator (which may be the ward sister) to develop and chair these sessions. There is a tendency for nurses to get so carried away with their detailed knowledge of the patient, that the relevant findings of that particular day related to the care plan are not presented.

## Nurse performance evaluation

Evaluation of the nursing care which patients are receiving can also be carried out by evaluating the nursing staff's performance. The introduction of the nursing process system of care demands new knowledge and skills which must be carried out at an acceptable level of competence. The ward sister or charge nurse, together with the member of staff or nurse learner concerned, must search for new ways of finding out if these goals are being reached. This involves both the learner and the teacher getting together and establishing learning and performance objectives. For example, while working on the unit/ward the learner or staff member will:

1. Utilise the components of the nursing process in giving care to patients during clinical practice. This is then graded according to the competence with which nursing histories, assessments, plan of care and progress notes have been written.

2. Communicate effectively with nurse colleagues and other members of the health-care team. This is graded according to how well the nurse has written down and passed on information, and presented her patient at a case conference and at physicians' ward rounds.

3. Evaluate the nursing care which has been given to her patient. This is graded by analysing the patient's care plan, looking at the objectives and expected outcomes which have been set, and the content of the progress notes.

The member of staff or learner is also encouraged to fill in a self-evaluation form which should include, in her own words, how well she feels she performed each of the following responsibilities (if possible, examples of competence should be given to illustrate points made):

(a) to patients;

(b) to other nurse colleagues (associate and primary nurses);

(c) to the ward sister;

(d) to the care co-ordinator if sister was off duty;

(e) to the medical staff;

(f) to paramedical staff;

(g) to self;

(h) to other departments.

The sister or charge nurse should also write a report based on these areas and the two should confer at an evaluation session, where new objectives of performance could be developed.

Audits of nurse competence in using the stages of the nursing process may be developed and used for self, peer or subordinate evaluation.

Ganong and Ganong (1977) developed a useful systematic approach to staff evaluation (*Figure 9.9*).

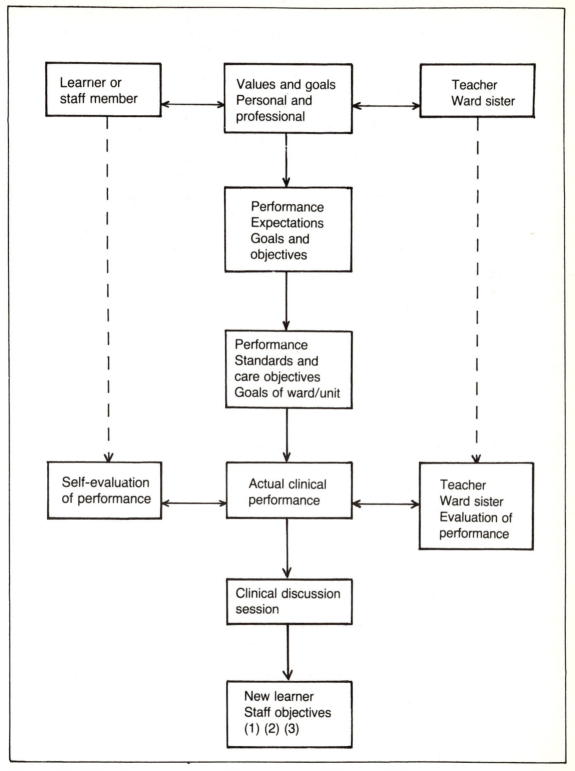

*Figure 9.9*  Self-evaluation flow chart (after Ganong and Ganong, 1977)

# Overcoming some common problems of using the nursing process

1. *Complicated assessment outlines.* In an enthusiastic endeavour to cover all the eventualities and likely alternatives which may crop up when taking a patient's nursing history, very long and complicated assessment outlines have been designed. When designing a nursing history format, start simply and build up the record. Keep it simple and easy to follow and do not let the paperwork get out of control. It is only there to act as a prompt and guide to the areas to be considered when carrying out the assessment.

2. *Too much emphasis on an interview.* Remember that information about a patient can be collected from many different sources (see Chapter 6 on Assessment). It has been assumed that, in all situations, an interview with the patient is the only method of data collection; this is not so.

3. *Physical examination and observation are not encouraged enough.* Remember always to make a thorough head-to-toe systematic observational assessment of the patient (see *Figure 4.2*). The emphasis is on observation of the patient's behaviour and bodily functions and should always be carried out discreetly and sympathetically (*Figure 9.10*).

4. *Does one need to possess special qualifications and skills to understand and carry out the nursing process?* There is need for practice and careful guidance through the stages of the nursing process with a trained nurse, in order to become proficient in its use. Some of the skills involved in the nursing process are easy; others will require continued advice from a teacher or expert nurse practitioner.

5. *Failure to clarify the patient's problems with him.* Remember the philosophy behind the nursing process – the patient should always be involved as far as possible. When you have assessed or evaluated a patient's progress try to involve him in the decisions which are made. It is his life not yours. There are times when you may disagree with an analysis of what his problems are. Such a disagreement must be carefully handled, so seek the advice of a tutor or clinical expert (*Figure 9.11*).

6. *Stating the patient's problems can be difficult.* Sometimes it is very difficult to state exactly what the patient's problem is. One helpful tip is to think of the nursing actions you are going to carry out — what you are going to do for this patient. Does he really need nursing help or assistance with his activities of daily living?

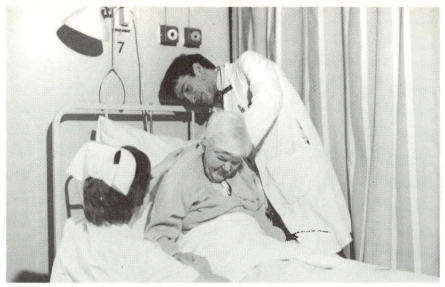

*Figure 9.10* 'Remember always to make a thorough head-to-toe systematic observational assessment of the patient.' If a good working relationship is developed with the doctor, this can be a joint effort

7. *Long- and short-term goals or expected outcomes.* There is a tendency in care plans to write ultimate goals of care or vague unrealistic outcomes of what the nurse or patient hopes will happen, rather than focus down on some measurable criteria which you can evaluate in stages to see if the patient has progressed or not (*Figure 9.12*).

8. *Problem-orientated charting is needed.* The nursing process is not a method of writing or designing a new form of nursing record. The way we record nursing actions with patients based on the nursing process approach should be recorded carefully, and problem-orientated charting is one of the best methods of achieving this (see Chapter 6).

9. *Evaluation methods need encouraging.* There is a tendency to focus on the assessment stage of the nursing process and virtually ignore the evaluation stage. This is unfortunate, as the evaluation stage is very important for determining just how effective nursing care has been. Always be thinking of methods which can be used to measure how good the nursing is and how well the patient has been cared for.

10. *Negative attitudes of staff.* One of the greatest difficulties in developing the nursing process approach in any nursing situation is the attitude and the commitment of both trained and untrained staff. There are many reasons for negative attitudes and resistance to change, some of which are based on insufficient knowledge of the nursing process, threat of the loss of power and authority, and an unwillingness to try something new.

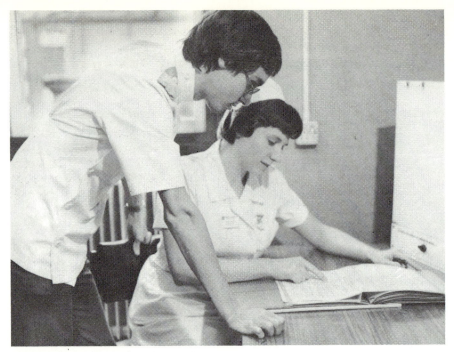

*Figure 9.11*   'Seek the advice of a tutor or clinical expert'

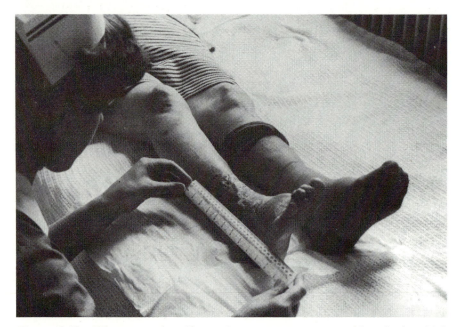

*Figure 9.12*   When assessing, 'focus down on some measurable criteria which you can evaluate'. Here, the nurse is seen measuring a leg ulcer

11. *Lack of support and advice.* Insufficient back-up and advice from both managers and teachers can lead to fragmentation and isolation. There is a need for good communication between nurse managers, practitioners and teachers. The appointment of a special nursing process co-ordinator/consultant may help to encourage this and offer expert advice for nurses trying to use the nursing process.

12. *Difficulty in maintaining enthusiasm.* If nurses do not receive adequate advice, support and help, enthusiasm may waver and a return to routinised nursing care result (*Figure 9.13*). The nursing process can motivate and stimulate those giving nursing care. Encourage, support and reward progress, however small. Be flexible and do not expect too much too soon.

13. *Creativity must be preserved.* Remember, the nursing process is orientated towards preserving the individuality of the patient. It should also be used in a creative way to reach that goal. This book only provides guidelines and principles for nursing application. You may discover better and more efficient ways of reaching the ideals of the nursing process.

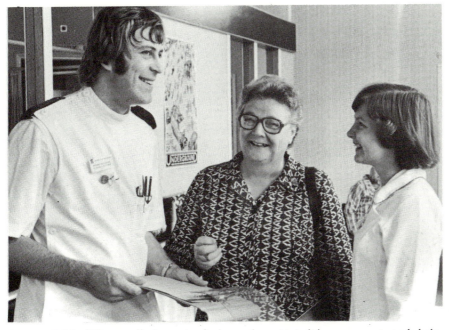

*Figure 9.13* 'If nurses do not receive adequate advice, support and help, enthusiasm may waver'

14. *Application demands a lot of energy, hard work and commitment.* There are few, if any, short cuts to becoming an expert in the nursing process. There is need for patience, as skills can be developed gradually.

15. *Levels and quality of staffing.* Extreme staff shortages will affect the application of the nursing process, but the education and response of staff members is just as important, if not more so. To some degree and in some way it should apply to the nursing process in any clinical nursing situation.

16. *Confidentiality.* Finally, patients generally have great respect for and trust in the nurse. When information about them is written down, the patient should know this and be assured that it will be used very, carefully and by nurses only. If the patient does not want something to be known or written, then his wishes must be respected.

# Appendix I

# An Actual Nursing Care Study using the Nursing Process

## Introduction

'The unique function of the nurse is to assist the individual, sick or well, in the performance of those activities contributing to health, or its recovery (or to peaceful death), that he would perform unaided if he had the necessary strength, will or knowledge, and to do this in such a way as to help him gain independence as rapidly as possible' (Henderson, 1966).

Virginia Henderson has put into words the overall aims and attitudes of the nurse as she carries out her individualised care for a patient, which is part of a team approach whose combined aim is to improve the quality of life.

The following is a descriptive account, by a student SRN, of an interview with a patient followed by the relevant nursing history format and care plans.

## Collection of information

Information was initially obtained from the patient, the female friend who accompanied her on admission, past medical records and observation of the general state of the patient shortly after admission to the geriatric assessment ward on 25th August, 1981. The nursing history took the pattern of an informal chat, by the bedside, where the patient could become accustomed to her new surroundings and the nurse–patient bonds begin to be established.

After I had introduced myself by name, the lady said that she preferred to be known as 'May', rather than Mrs . . . , and she readily volunteered the following information.

She was a Tonbridge person and had been so all of her life — she would be 85 years old on 10th November, 1981. May's admission had been planned through referral by her general practitioner to the geriatric assessment ward consultant because of what she understood was a left-leg thrombosis. She accepted that her condition necessitated admission to hospital, but admitted that this caused her husband much anxiety. He was not present with May on arrival at the ward, because she had advised him to stay at home.

May had been a housewife all her life and had one son, whom they often visit in Scotland. He was contactable on the telephone, but May was reluctant to cause him any undue concern about her condition. Her present state of health had not required them to need the social services. She found the Church of England beliefs and practices beneficial but was not a regular churchgoer. She did enjoy walking and felt that this may have caused her present condition.

During the past she suffered from peritonitis 'years ago' and at that time developed a thrombosis of the left leg. Since then she has had problems with recurrent left-leg pain, a left-ankle ulcer four years ago, a miscarriage and right-hip and left-hand arthritis.

On examination she appeared to be generally in a good condition. Her hair was short, grey and well kept. She used two pairs of glasses, but on later observation it was clear she preferred to wear them as little as possible. There was a mild hearing defect for which she had an aid, worn infrequently. The mouth state was good — no evidence of ulcers, coated tongue or infections. Upper and lower teeth dentures were worn 24 hours a day and only removed for cleaning purposes. Her respiratory function was good and she was a non-smoker. There was evidence of nocturnal urgency of micturition. She found that often it was necessary to pass urine three times during the night. During the day she had noticed no frequency. Elimination of faeces took place regularly once daily.

Her skin appeared hydrated, intact, pink and warm over the whole of her body except for the area of her left leg. This was swollen, hard, pink/bluish in colour and cool to the touch. Her calf measured 36 cms (5 cms from the patella) and the thigh = 56 cms (16 cms from the upper portion of the patella). The patient noticed a throbbing sensation in her left leg, but it gave her no pain. The ulcer on the inner aspect of her left leg was 1 in. by $1\frac{1}{2}$ in.; it appeared to be a small superficial ulcer developed on the site of the larger ulcer present four years ago. May treated this with zinc and lint dressings. Both heels were intact. There was evidence of dry skin on her right leg. During the past three weeks she had only been able to mobilise to the bathroom, but had practised her leg exercises in order to keep herself mobile. Normally she was a very active cheerful woman who enjoyed visiting friends, walking and shopping. Her sleeping pattern over the past three weeks had been good, and no sedation has been required. Her dietary habits of late had been poor, due to feeling nauseated. She had been able to carry out her own hygiene needs with slight help from her husband, and enjoyed a good thorough daily wash. Her husband also helped her to dress.

Recordings were taken of her vital signs in order to establish a baseline. The blood pressure was 206/120, pulse 68 beats per minute and temperature 36.7°C. Her urine sample showed no evidence of the presence of ketones, blood protein or glucose and was pH 6. She weighed 63.5 kgs on admission.

Further information was gained from an informal talk with May's friend who accompanied her on admission to hospital. The friend lived about seven miles from May and was contactable on the phone. She admitted that May's left leg had been swollen and painful for three weeks, causing her to be unable to mobilise. This condition was quite obviously causing distress to both husband and wife, although the friend felt that they tried to cover up their anxieties. The friend felt that May would be able to adapt well to the hospital environment and proved to be an excellent objective source of information about May's home conditions.

May lived with her husband in an old-fashioned terraced house, three rooms upstairs and three downstairs. It was not modernised, but kept in good condition. During the past three weeks May had used the settee in the lounge as her bed, going upstairs to the bathroom. They had a 'wash-house' outside the house which May used throughout the year, with two commodes for their use when needed.

Throughout the informal chat, May showed a determined, cheerful, outgoing type of personality. Her friend informed me that May wished only to live for a few more years 'to put everything right', and therefore had made up her mind to recover. May was well spoken and tended to under-emphasise her condition, due to an anxious husband.

On referral to May's medical notes she was diagnosed as having an ileo femoral thrombosis and the proposed medical scheme of treatment was for oral anticoagulation.

# Assessment

On the basis of the information collected about May, a general assessment of her physical, social and psychological state was made, so that potential and real problems of nursing the patient could be identified and a plan of nursing care established to meet these problems.

Physically, May appeared to be in reasonable condition. The main identifiable problem was of her swollen and numb left leg and the ankle ulcer thereon. Her appetite appeared to be affected by this condition, which caused frequent bouts of nausea. Mobility had been affected and with a struggle she was able to walk. She was unable to care for all of her hygiene needs or dress fully unaided, stressing the fact that her left leg resulted in decreased ability.

Normally, May was an active woman. Of late she had spent most of her time resting on the lounge settee; this posed a potential problem of lung congestion, but there was no evidence of any respiratory disorder on admission.

She appeared to be mildly over-weight on admission, possibly due to lack of mobility. Her vital signs on admission showed evidence of hypertension, when her blood pressure was taken at rest. This could have been due to anxiety, being over-weight and the fact that blood pressure rises with age, and therefore may only have been a transient increase.

Normally, May had no problems of micturition, but there was evidence recently of urgency at night. This was causing her a restless night's sleep, although no sedation was being taken.

When fit and healthy, May was able to visit friends, and go shopping and walking, but due to the immobilisation of her left leg she had been unable to carry out her normal social habits. She appeared the type of woman to self-treat the symptoms of ill health until they became too severe. She was determined to regain full health and took a very practical and realistic view of her disabilities.

Initially, May was assessed on her physical fitness, ability to move, activity, incontinence and mental state. On the Knoll scale she scored 7 points.

# Plan of nursing care

The first and most important problem identified through an assessment of May's condition was her immobility. It was expected that as the symptoms of her deep vein thrombosis decreased under medical treatment she would have an increase in mobility. To reach this aim she was to remain on bed rest during the first two days in hospital, then practise non-weight-bearing movements from bed to chair to commode, for the left leg, and from admission to practise right-leg exercises.

Due to the fact that she would be spending her first two days resting in bed and exercising her right leg only, there was a potential problem of pressure sore development on the right heel and buttocks. Also, there was a history of right-hip arthritis which may have caused further immobilisation. In order to prevent pressure sore development, May was to be encouraged to transfer her weight from side to back to side while in bed. Her skin was also to be checked daily in order to make sure no cracks developed in the skin surface.

On admission, there was evidence of hypertension in the blood pressure recording; therefore this, along with the heart rate, was measured four hourly initially. The temperature was also taken four hourly to check for a pyrexia which may be present in deep vein thrombosis development. These recordings were to be charted and any irregular developments or changes to be reported in order to maintain stable vital signs.

May did not complain of left-leg pain or headaches as a side-effect of hypertension, but her strong-willed character may have overridden any desire for analgesia. Potential pain was a problem; our aim was to relieve and prevent this. A bed-cradle was inserted to relieve the weight of the bed-clothes from her legs and analgesia was to be offered regularly and given if required.

The oedema of the left leg, as shown by the measurements on admission, was gross when compared to the observation of the right-leg size. In order to relieve the oedema, an input and output chart was to be used in order to check for an increased loss of water, indicating a reduction of oedema. Daily measurements of the thigh and calf were taken and a TED (thrombo-embolitic deterrent) elastic stocking worn to help the venous return of blood from the leg. The base end of her bed was elevated approximately 12 in. to help the flow of blood back to the heart, and when sitting out she was to use a stool.

May complained of eating small amounts over the last three weeks and at times feeling nauseated. Our aim was to increase her appetite and give her adequate nutrition. In order to reach our aim, her dietary input was observed and recorded, and small attractive portions were served. She was also encouraged to take some of her favourite drink of Guinness before meal times.

As a result of her lack of mobility and reduced activity, May had the potential problem of insufficient daily hygiene and lack of ability to dress. Our aim was to enable her to perform all self-care. Therefore it was planned initially to observe and report her ability when carrying out personal hygiene and changing clothes. If needed, one nurse would help to wash the lower half of her body and help with dressing.

There was evidence of nocturnal urgency of micturition which we aimed to relieve by first of all observing and reporting times at which the patient required toileting, and providing the commode four hourly until these times were established.

Lying in bed with legs elevated and only exercising her right leg posed the potential problem of lung congestion. To prevent this, May was to be encouraged to practise deep-breathing exercises to expand all lobes of her lungs and she was to be advised to sit upright when in bed.

The superficial left-ankle ulcer of the inner aspect of the foot had been present for a few weeks. The aim was to render her skin intact, with no breaks, and to achieve this the ulcer was cleaned and re-dressed daily, with reports of observation to be made in the Kardex.

There was some dry skin down the length of her right leg; therefore, in order to prevent any skin breakdown, olive oil was applied giving moisture to the skin.

May was slightly over-weight on admission, although she claimed to have been much heavier in recent years. Her body would benefit from a further reduction in weight. The dietician was therefore to be contacted and a reducing diet ordered. To monitor weight loss, May was weighed twice weekly.

## Implementation and evaluation

During this part of May's individualised nursing care, continued reassessments were made of her progress and new plans made to cater for this and any new problems which arose.

After two days of bed rest, during which time she was encouraged by the nurses to exercise her right leg, May was able to begin transferring herself from bed to chair to commode. By her fifth day in hospital she was mobilising with the aid of a TED stocking. On day nine a reassessment was made of her progress. She was by now walking to the table for meals unaided. She only appeared to find the left leg stiff and became tired easily if walking too much during the day. This problem was discontinued on the sixth day of hospitalisation.

The potential problem of pressure sores was reassessed daily, and after six days discontinued. Her skin remained intact, no breaks developed as she practised moving her weight regularly from side to back to side, and after a few days she was beginning to mobilise. May required a little reminding to move her weight when on bed rest.

Observations of her blood pressure four hourly showed it had stabilised and could therefore be discontinued after two days. Her pulse rate and temperature were monitored for a further five days due to slight fluctuations, but on a daily basis were normally taken at 2.00 p.m. No significant changes occurred in the vital signs and they stabilised and could therefore be discontinued.

The use of a bed-cradle at night to relieve the weight of the bed-clothes proved beneficial to May. She required no analgesia for the oedematous left leg, but the ulcer did cause a certain amount of discomfort on the tenth day, and analgesia was given according to the plan.

Initially, all the input and output were charted to check for a fluid loss, but this was discontinued on the sixth day as it produced very little indication as to her progress. The daily measurements of thigh and calf proved a beneficial measurement of reduction of oedema. By the ninth day her thigh had reduced by 3.5 cms in size and her calf decreased by 0.5 cms. The TED stocking was applied in the mornings and removed at night. Initially, help was given when the stocking was applied, and gradually under observation and instruction May managed to apply this stocking herself. The elevated base end of her bed proved to be beneficial in helping the drainage of fluid. On her second day, May complained of a burning sensation behind the kneecap, but this disappeared with the help of leg exercises.

It was observed that May ate very small amounts. Gradually, through serving small portions and appetising food, she began to take the reducing diet very well.

Assessment of May's ability to wash and dress showed that she could manage well attending to the top half of her body, but required help in washing her legs. She was aided with a full wash each day, as she expressed her feelings that a daily wash was essential. By the third day she was able to care for all of her own hygiene and was only aided when she desired a bath. This problem was discontinued on the sixth day.

There was no evidence from the night reports of nocturnal urgency of micturition. The commode was provided when needed, otherwise May was observed to have slept well.

The potential problem of lung congestion was avoided successfully following the plan of care and was discontinued after the sixth day.

Daily observation, cleaning and re-dressing of the superficial left-ankle ulcer showed little change in its state and by the ninth day a small break was developing below the original ulcer, which was 1 in. by $\frac{1}{2}$ in. in size. The dry skin on her right leg improved to healthy skin after a week and a half of daily applications of olive oil.

May's problem of being over-weight improved during the first nine days in hospital.

On the ninth day of her hospital stay it was decided on the ward round, by the team, in consultation with May, to continue her plan of care with the outlook of returning home in a week or so. This decision posed the potential problem of her ability to cope physically when returned home. The aim was to provide adequate support and preparation before departure. To achieve this it was planned to gradually introduce the idea of leaving hospital to allow May to carry out her normal routine during the day within the hospital setting, and a home visit was arranged with the ward occupational therapist to assess home facilities.

*Figures A.1–A.3* show the completed forms for May's nursing history, care plan and progress notes.

## Transfer home care plan

Before the home visit was undertaken, a further assessment of May's health was made in order to form a plan of care for her eventual transfer home. It was important that real and potential problems were identified before going on a home visit, so that her abilities within the home setting could be assessed.

The most important potential problem identified was that of a lack of mobility around her home due to the remaining left-leg oedema. It was therefore planned that her mobility should be observed and assessed when ascending and descending stairs, both inside and outside of the house, when moving around the house generally and when climbing in and out of the bath.

May's second potential problem on return home was that of exhaustion due to her determined and strong-willed frame of mind. The planned care was to observe and assess May with her husband, in the home surroundings, and to talk with them about the importance of a period of convalescence on returning home. The objectives were reinforced on return to hospital after the home visit.

On discharge from hospital to home, May had a potential problem of confusion with the tablets which she would be taking for anticoagulation. It was therefore decided to talk with May and her husband about the drug, its dose and how often it was to be taken, so that there was a clear understanding of the present medication. The importance of attending the anticoagulant clinic was also to be discussed.

| Jones | May |
|-------|-----|
| Surname | Forename(s) |

| Address: 30, View Close, Tonbridge, Kent | |
|---|---|

| Next of Kin: Husband — Albert Jones | Date of Birth: 10/11/1896 |
| | Age: 84 |

| Likes to be referred to as: May | Relevant Tel. Nos. Mrs Brooks (friend) (and next door neighbour) 1422 4311 |

| Date of Admission to Hospital: 25/8/81 | Ward: M 5 |

General Practitioner: Dr. Colenso, The Surgery: 4, Long Lane, Tonbridge, Kent

Reason for Admission: Assessment and possible anticoagulant therapy

Medical Diagnosis: Left Ileo-Femoral Thrombosis

Consultant: Dr. Brown

What Patient or Family understands about his/her condition:

Patient:- accepts diagnosis
Friend :- says Mrs Jones has had painful leg for over 3 weeks which has prevented her walking and caused much distress to both her and her husband.

Patient's and/or Family Reaction to Hospital Admission:

Patient:- does not mind being admitted to hospital but is aware of husband's anxiety over her condition.

Home Conditions: Friend = objective view. "Old fashioned terraced house", 3 up 3 down. Not modernised. Kept in good condition. During past three weeks patient has used the settee in lounge to sleep on. Wash house-outside- which patient still uses. 2 commodes - toilet outside. Bathroom upstairs.

*Figure A.1*    Nursing history — taken from patient and meaningful friend

| History taken from | |
|---|---|
| Patient and friend | |
| | Record No. **72177** |

Meaningful Person in Life:                                        Significant others/pets:

Mrs Brooks - close friend and neighbour
Son - Jack Jones

Community Resources (D.N.H.V., Social Worker, Meals on Wheels etc. . . .):

None

General Health History & Previous Hospital Admission:

Peritonitis "Years ago".
Recurrent left leg pain
Left leg ulcer on ankle - 4 years ago.
Right hip and right and left hand (arthritis) - past 20 years

Religious Practices or Beliefs Patient finds helpful:
C/E

Recreational Activities and Past/Present Work Life:
Housewife - walking, reading, sewing

General Assessment on Admission: Hair: - kept in good condition. Eyes: - uses spectacles for reading
and general day. Ears: - mild hearing defect - uses hearing aid. Mouth: - good buccal state -
wears dentures. Respiratory function: - good, no problems. Micturition: - nocturnal urgency x 3,
no complaints of frequency. Elimination: - regularly once per day. Skin: - hydrated, no pressure
sores. Left leg swollen and hard, colour - pink/bluish - cool to touch. Complains of "throbbing
sensation" in leg. No severe pain. Ulcer on inner aspect of left ankle 1" x ½".
Mobility: - for past three weeks walking restricted to house. Activity: - normally very active
cheerful lady, also enjoys visiting friends, walking and shopping. Sleeping: - over past 3
weeks, slept well, no sedation taken. Diet: - for past three weeks - mildly nauseated, otherwise
small amount of food taken. Hygiene: - enjoys daily wash. Copes with most of own needs.
Dressing: - requires help of husband. Observations: - B.P. 200/120  P.68  T.36  Knoll scale = 7
Urinalysis - N.A.D.  pH 6  Weight  63.5kgs.

*N.B.*   Note the name of the person who carried out the assessment and if patient or relative or both
involved

| Signature  D. Hosegood | Date 25·8·81 |
|---|---|

*Figure A.1*    continued

**May Jones**    72177

CARE PLAN

| Date Commenced | Patient's Nursing Problem | Expected Outcome | Nursing Care Plan | Tick when completed Date/Time Discontinued | Signature |
|---|---|---|---|---|---|
| 25/8/81 | 1) Immobilisation due to physical condition. | 1) Increase in mobility as symptoms decrease during treatment of DVT. | 1)(a) Non weight bearing left leg. (b) Bedrest for 2 days. Op 27/8/81. (c) Encourage ph. to exercise R. leg. | 1/9/81 | R. Whittle |
| 25/8/81 | 2) Potential problems of pressure sores due to condition of left leg. | 2) Prevention of pressure sore development. | 2)(a) Weight transferred side - back - side when in bed. (b) Check daily skin state. | 1/9/81 | R. Whittle |
| 25/8/81 | 3)(Vital signs.) Potential problem of deterioration in medical condition. | 3) Stable vital signs T-36 P-68. | 3)(a) Daily observation of T.P. & B.P. (b) Chart and report significant changes. | 3/9/81 | R. Whittle |
| 25/8/81 | 4) Pain in left leg. | 4) Adequate pain relief, patient expresses satisfaction with analgesics used. | 4)(a) Bed cradle to relieve weight on swollen left leg. (b) Regular analgesics as required. | 1/9/81 | R. Whittle |
| 25/8/81 | 5) Oedema of left leg, see measurements in cms, due to deep vein thrombosis. | 5) Reduction of oedema by 5 cms. | 5)(a) All input and output to be charted. (b) Daily measurement of thigh and calf. (c) TED stocking and elevate end of bed. (d) Elevate leg when sitting out. | | |
| 25/8/81 | 6) Low dietary intake, with potential problem of increasing loss of weight. | 6) Increase appetite if possible, and maintain weight at 11st lbs. | 6)(a) Observe and record diet intake. (b) Serve attractive small portions of food to patient. | | |
| 25/8/81 | 7) Difficulty in maintaining hygiene and ability to dress self. | 7) Ability to perform all self-care. | 7)(a) Observe patient ability when carrying out personal hygiene and changing clothes. (b) Aid of one nurse when washing lower half of body and dressing. | 3/9/81 | R. Whittle |

*Figure A.2*   Nursing care plan

## May Jones    72177

CARE PLAN

| Date Commenced | Patient's Nursing Problem | Expected Outcome | Nursing Care Plan | Tick when completed Date/Time Discontinued | Signature |
|---|---|---|---|---|---|
| 25/8/81 | 8) Nocturnal urgency of micturition. | 8) Relief of urgency. | 8)(a) Observe times at which patient requires toileting. (b) Provide commode 4 hrly during night. | | |
| 25/8/81 | ~~9) Potential problem of lung congestion~~ | ~~9) Prevention of lung congestion with good intake of air and expiration.~~ | 9) (a) Encourage deep breathing exercises to expand lungs. (b) Encourage patient to sit upright in bed. | 1/9/81 | R. Whittle |
| 25/8/81 | ~~10) Potential problem of side-effects of hypertension.~~ | 10) Stable vital signs — 180/100 | 10) (a) Monitor and chart B.P. daily. (b) Report significant changes to medical staff. | 3/9/81 | R. Whittle |
| 25/8/81 | 11) Superficial left ankle ulcer 1½" x 1" and 1" x ½". | 11) (a) Reduction in size. (b) Skin intact, no further breakdown. | 11) (a) Daily observation and record progress of wound breakdown. (b) Clean and redress wound daily with Savlodil and dry dressing. | | |
| 25/8/81 | 12) Dry skin on right leg. | 12) Moist healthy skin. | 12) Apply olive oil to leg daily. | | |
| 3/9/81 | 13) Ability to cope with self-care activities on return home. | 13) (a) Adequate support and preparation for return home. (b) Patient expresses satisfaction over transfer home. | 13) (a) Introduce idea of leaving hospital on set date. (b) Assess patient's self-care activities and carry out a home visit with her. (c) Contact support services and district nurse. | | |
| 3/9/81 | 14) Potential problem of bleeding due to anticoagulant therapy. | 14) (a) No signs of bleeding. (b) Patient aware of dangers. | 14) (a) Observe for signs of bleeding and bruising — test urine daily. Check faeces. (b) Teach patient. | | |

*Figure A.2*    continued

PART OF PATIENT'S PROGRESS NOTES

Name.... **May Jones** ........

Hospital No.... **72177** .......

| Date.......... | |
|---|---|
| 25/8/81 | Admitted at 4.30 p.m. with friend, Mrs Brooks. This lady appears very cheerful, keen to sort out her problems and return home. Well spoken woman tending to under-emphasise her condition due to an anxious husband, whom she would not be surprised if he did not visit her in hospital. REASON FOR ADMISSION – Swollen left leg. On examination the left leg was hard and pink/bluish in colour. Measurements – Calf – 36 cms (5 cm from patella), thighs – 56 cms (16 cm from upper part of patella). Also on left ankle, inner aspect, an ulcer 1" x 1½" to which she applied zinc and lint dressings. Both heels are intact.<br>              – D. Hosegood (Student Nurse) |
| 27/8/81 | Late to settle 11 p.m. but says she "slept well." No change in care plan during the night – C. Jones (Staff Nurse) |
| 25/8/81<br>10 a.m. | Ward Round TED stocking and foam wedge if available, and use tipping bed for rectal examination to exclude pelvic compression of circulation. Also ask Rheumatologist to see knee to exclude arthritis origin of inflammation. Probable diagnosis DVT. Continue with anticoagulants. Mobilise gently with TED stockings. Legs elevated when at rest. Please measure legs as instructed on care plan.<br>              – R. Whittle (Primary Nurse) |
| 28/8/81<br>2 p.m. | 1) Patient transferring well from bed to commode. 2) Skin intact, moving position well in bed. 3) B.P = 174/80, T = 38°C, P = 68. 8.P. lowered since admission. 4) No analgesia required. 5) Input and output satisfactory. Calf 33 cm, thigh 52 cm. Patient complains of "burning" feeling behind kneecap. Left leg appears less solid. TED stocking to be applied to left leg and bed to be elevated to aid drainage of fluid. 6) Taking small amount of diet. 7) Managed to wash all of body apart from left leg. 8) Encouraged to sit upright in bed and expand lungs. Appears slightly breathless on exertion. 9) B.P. at 10 a.m. down to 174/80. 10) Cleaned with Savodil and dressed with Melolin. Wound appears to be oozing small amounts of fluid. 11) Olive oil applied. 12) To be weighed this afternoon – 140 lb.<br>              – D. Hosegood (Student Nurse) |
| 28/8/81<br>Night Report | Up to commode once in night, otherwise no change in care plan. Says she slept well from about 10 p.m.<br>              – M.Beeming (S.E.N.) |

*Figure A.3* Progress notes

PART OF PATIENT'S PROGRESS NOTES

Name... May Jones

Hospital No... 72.177

| Date | |
|---|---|
| 29/8/81 2 p.m. | 1) Remains on bed rest. 3) and 9) Pulse and temp. stable. B.P. quite high 180/120 at 2 p.m. seen by Dr Kay, no change in treatment at present – continue care plan. 4) No complaints of pain. 5) Calf 34 cms, thigh 59 cms. 7) Washed herself in bed without any difficulty. 11) Dressing to be carried out and reported later. |
| | — R. Whittle (Primary Nurse) |
| (A few days later) | |
| 3/9/81 | Re-assessment of Patient. |
| | Knoll Score – 8 |
| | 5) Oedema of left leg remains unchanged since 1/9/81. Calf 36·5 cms, thigh 52·5 cms. Patient finds difficulty when applying TED stocking over left foot but can manage to pull the stocking up once past the ankle. She requires observation and instruction as to the correct method of application. She continues to elevate left leg when out of bed. 6) Taking small amount of diet: appears to be enjoying her meals. 11) Ulcer redressed this morning, small break in skin noticed below original ulcer, approximately 1" x ½". 12) Olive oil had good effect on dry skin on right leg, patient continues to use lotion. 6) Weighed today – 65·4 kgs, increase of 1·9 kgs since admission. 13) Patient encouraged to care for her own hygiene this morning and when getting in and out of bath she managed well. She appears to monitor her activity well according to how tired she feels. |
| | — D. Hosegood (Student Nurse) |

*Figure A.3*  continued

The fourth potential problem identified was that of the possible recurrence of her symptoms of swelling, numbness and throbbing in the left leg, on return home. In order to allay any fears of this kind, advice and reassurance was to be given, during the home visit, to both May and her husband and assurance given that their general practitioner would be keeping in close contact with them.

The home visit was carried out by the occupational therapist, primary nurse and district nurse on the fifteenth day of May's hospitalisation. It proved to be a beneficial event. The identified potential problem of a lack of mobility around the home was discontinued as May could descend and ascend the stairs, inside and outside the house, with relative ease. It was decided to contact the social services in order to provide a hand-rail outside the back door, by the steps, to facilitate an easier access to the outside wash-house. May managed fairly well when climbing in and out of the bath, but it was felt that with the aid of a bath-rail attached to the taps she could manage with greater ease and safety.

The potential problem of exhaustion was clearly possible when May was assessed in her home surroundings. She was therefore firmly advised to take a period of convalescence on return home before gradually increasing her activities.

May showed that she had a clear understanding of her drug therapy and this potential problem could be discontinued.

Advice was given about the possible recurrence of a deep vein thrombosis and the action necessary if the symptoms developed. This was clearly understood by May and her husband and the 'potential problem' could be discontinued on the chart.

On return to hospital these findings were evaluated with May and the hospital care team, in conjunction with the district nurse, decided that the original condition for which May was admitted to hospital was greatly improved and she appeared capable in her home surroundings. By the seventeenth day of her hospitalisation the remaining 'real' and 'potential' problems of her condition were discontinued on the chart. She was now ready for the transfer home into the community services of her general practitioner, district nurse and the Social Services Department.

*Figure A.4* shows May's transfer care plan.

TRANSFER CARE PLAN

| Date Commenced | Patient's Nursing Problem | Expected Outcome | Nursing Care Plan | Tick when completed Date/Time Discontinued | Signature |
|---|---|---|---|---|---|
| 8/9/81 Before home visit | 1) Potential problem of lack of sufficient mobility around home due to physical problem in the left leg. | 1) Mobilised well upstairs. 2) Mobilised well outside. | Observe and assess ability of patient: 1) Mounting and descending stairs around house. 2) Mobilising around house. 3) Descending stairs outside house and into wash house. 4) Ability getting in and out of bath. | | |
| | 2) Exhaustion on return home, due to increased effect of mobility and movement | 2) Gradual increase of involvement in daily routine. | 1) Observe and assess in home surroundings 2) Talk with patient and husband about the period of convalescence after being in hospital. 3) Reinforce objective on return to hospital. 4) Encourage patient on return to hospital to carry out as much of her normal daily routine as possible within the hospital setting. | | |
| | 3) Potential problem of confusion with tablets due to ignorance of side-effects of drugs. | 3) Clear understanding of drug regime (patient verbalises this without prompting) | 1) Talk with patient and husband about drugs on return home. 2) Explain prescription and reason for attending Anticoagulant Clinic. | | |
| | 4) Potential problem of recurrence of DVT (deep vein thrombosis), due to immobility. | 4) Adequate advice and reassurance as to possibility of DVT recurrence (patient verbalises awareness of the side-effects of bed rest and immobility). | 1) Talk with patient and husband about causes of DVT. 2) Advise on rest, relaxation and exercise. | | |

*Figure A.4*  Transfer care plan

# Appendix II

# Assessment of Confusion*

## Abbreviated mental test score

Score 1 for each correct answer (if patient scores below 7, then confusion is present).

*Ask patient:*

1. Age

2. Time (to nearest hour).

3. Address (for recall at end of test; this should be repeated by the patient to ensure that it has been heard correctly).

4. Year.

5. Name of hospital.

6. Recognition of 2 persons (e.g. Doctor/Nurse).

7. Date of birth.

8. Year of First World War.

9. Name of present monarch.

10. Count backwards — 20–1
    or
    Count backwards names of months in a year — December–January.

---

* Developed by Dr R. Gaind (Guy's Hospital, 1981).

# Appendix III

# Student Exercises

## Exercise 1: Identification of patient problems

Read the following passages taken from a case study and try to identify the
nursing problems — actual and potential — which the patient is facing:

David, aged 22 years, was admitted to hospital suffering from a severe heart
complaint (aortic valve incompetence), complicated by infective
endocarditis.

Shortly after his admission, David's condition deteriorated and he became
very lethargic and unwilling to wash himself. When lying down in bed, he
found that he was becoming very breathless, but this was relieved when he
sat upright, supported by pillows. At the same time, frothy sputum was
becoming troublesome and this was reluctantly coughed up on occasions.
There was also the difficulty of movement while in bed, and David rarely
moved his legs or changed his position, which meant that there was the
possibility that he would develop a deep vein thrombosis in his ankles and
legs. At times, David found that he was having difficulty in passing urine.

Due to the accumulation of these difficulties, David become very annoyed
and appeared to resent the way the nurses tried to do things for him which
previously he had no difficulty in doing by himself. Meal-times were greeted
with disinterest and he rarely ate the food which was prepared for him. He
took fluids fairly well, however, but because of his poor diet he complained of
constipation. The large amounts of antibiotics given intramuscularly twice
daily also caused David much discomfort, but the doctors were very
reluctant to change to intravenous administration because of the risk of
infection by this route.

As previously mentioned, the oedema which involved David's ankles and
legs was forming in other parts of his body and the response to the prescribed
diuretic was questioned.

*Now that you have read this:*

1. Try to write down the nursing problems which the patient is facing; for
   example: (1) David's difficulty in maintaining his own personal state of
   hygiene and comfort.
   *Note:* There are at least 9 other problems which you should be able to
   distinguish.

2. Write down the 'potential' nursing problems which the patient is facing; for example: There are at least 3 other potential nursing problems besides pressure sores and deep vein thrombosis.

## Possible answers

*Suggested identification of problems which David is facing:*

1. Difficulty in maintaining his own personal state of hygiene and comfort.

2. Lethargic emotional state.

3. Difficulty in breathing unless in an upright position.

4. Difficulty in expectorating frothy sputum.

5. Difficulty in moving in bed due to his oedema, mental state and general condition.

6. Difficulty in passing urine.

7. Emotional reaction to his illness and deteriorating condition.

8. Difficulty in maintaining his own nutritional state.

9. Change in bowel habits and development of constipation.

10. Emotional reaction to his medical treatment, following the pain which this is causing him.

*Potential problems faced by David include:*

1. Pressure sores.

2. Painful swollen legs due to deep vein thrombosis.

3. Lung congestion due to a chest infection.

4. Malnutrition.

5. Fluid and electrolyte imbalance.

# Exercise 2

On consultation with a tutor, you may now feel that you are ready to make an assessment of a patient in the clinical setting in which you work.

Using the nursing history format or ideas outlined in this book, design your own nursing assessment form and then obtain the relevant information. Classify it and then determine the nursing problems of the patient.

Discuss your findings with a colleague and/or your tutor.

# Exercise 3

Use the problems you identified with the patient in Exercise 1 and identify the expected outcomes of nursing care; then suggest appropriate nursing plans/actions.
Reproduce this work using the following three headings:

| Patient's problems | Expected outcomes | Plan of care |
|---|---|---|
|  |  |  |

Remember, expected outcomes should explain the behaviour you expect the patient to exhibit.
Do this exercise alone initially, then consult a colleague and/or your tutor.

# Exercise 4: The case conference

Organise a conference of persons concerned in the care of a patient for whom you have used the nursing process approach. Present to them the assessment made, the plan of care and the patient outcomes.
By discussion, evaluate your performance at each stage of the process; then list any changes you would now make in the plan of care and your reason for doing so.

# Exercise 5

Obtain copies of completed nursing records/Kardex used in your clinical area.
Go through these critically, bearing the following questions in mind:

1. Is there evidence that a nursing assessment has been made?

2. Is there a list of the patient's problems?

3. Is there a plan of nursing care identified for each problem?

4. Are expected outcomes present and do they relate to specific short-term behaviour rather than longer term goals of care?

5. What is the quality of the progress report writing? For example, is it readable?

6. Can you gain an insight into the progress which the patient is making from reading the records?

7. Are all entries on the notes dated and signed properly?

8. How many abbreviations are used?

9. Is there any evidence that periodic evaluations have been made of the patient's progress?

10. Have nursing observations been recorded relating to both physical and emotional nursing care interventions?

11. Are there too many subjective nursing conclusions? For example, 'good day', 'satisfactory', 'good night'.

12. Have there been any crossings-out or mistakes made which have not been deleted correctly?

# Exercise 6

Using the following headings of a process recording sheet, encourage students either to get together with an agreeable partner or with a patient, and then talk to each other for about 45 minutes:

| What the patient or colleague communicates verbally and non-verbally | What the nurse communicates verbally and non-verbally | Perceptions of or about the patient or colleague | Thoughts and/ or feelings about these perceptions |
|---|---|---|---|
| | | | |

Students should then write up their work and discuss it with another colleague and/or tutor. Reasons for perceptions, thoughts and feelings of the student during the interaction and communication skills should be the main focus of these discussions.

# Exercise 7: Videotape simulation

The use of videotape simulation is a most effective way of helping students learn about themselves and their social skills. Students are selected to play the role of interviewer and interviewee. Each is then given instructions as to the role she is to play. For example:

SITUATION
*Patient:* Miss Wynnifred Jones

You have been admitted to a geriatric assessment unit for investigations of weight loss, incontinence and treatment of leg ulcers.

Recently, unknown to you, your behaviour has become rather 'strange' (i.e. you do not like going to bed, changing your clothes or speaking to strangers). With very careful persuasion, a district nurse who you are fond of and who has looked after you for years, has suggested that you should come into hospital for investigations and treatment (she, in fact, brought you in!). You are continually hungry and thirsty and look on hospital as a place where you will hopefully meet people and find a bit of life! Unfortunately, so far the place looks dead and the people in it 'geriatric'.

This is not the place for you and you would like to go home as soon as possible. On this second day of your admission a nurse who you think you like but are still unsure, has come to speak to you. You have seen some improvement in your condition and 'they' (i.e. the doctors) have told you that you have diabetes (unfortunately you do not know what that means). You feel that you would be better off at home.

SITUATION
*Nurse:* Eunice Leeming

You have been in nursing for longer than you care to remember. An old lady with a behavioural problem and recently diagnosed diabetes is no real problem on the surface. But you are wise enough to know that this lady is a particularly delicate patient who requires careful handling.

Yesterday she was brought in by *her* district nurse and you have let her settle in. Now, a day later, you feel it would be a good opportunity to interview her. Medical treatment for the diabetes was started yesterday with insulin and continues with tablets. Her ulcers need careful attention, and you suspect she is incontinent but are not sure.

The night staff have told you that Miss Wynnifred Jones did not sleep in her bed last night and refuses to change her clothes.

# Some essay questions for further study and thought

1. Select a patient whom you have nursed in a hospital ward and devise a nursing care plan to cover a 48-hour period during his/her stay.
2. After assessing a patient, what would lead you to suspect that a problem of dehydration existed? Discuss the nursing actions that may be implemented to assist the patient to overcome this problem.

3. Discuss the problems you have encountered in attempting to use the nursing process in caring for patients in a particular clinical setting. How might these problems be resolved?

4. Compare and discuss the problems you have encountered in attempting to use the nursing process either in the community compared to hospital or in acute medical/surgical wards compared to longer stay clinical areas. Suggest ways in which these problems can be resolved.

5. Explain the difference between long-term and short-term expected outcomes in planning a patient's nursing care.

6. Take one common problem of a patient admitted to hospital for either medical or surgical treatment, and describe the care you would give in relation to this problem, the rationale for the care and how you would evaluate its effectiveness.

7. What principles would you use in changing the organisation of a ward from task-orientated to individualised patient care?

8. What do you consider to be the advantages of using the nursing process in the care of the elderly sick person?

9. Select one clinical nursing research study. Discuss the means by which the findings from this study may be used to modify nursing practice.

10. Discuss the following statement: 'The more you can learn about yourself, the better you will be at finding out information about the patient.'

# Appendix IV

# United Kingdom Reading List on the Nursing Process

## Books and booklets

Hunt, J.M. and Marks-Maran, D.J., *Nursing Care Plans: The Nursing Process at Work*, Aylesbury, H.M. & M. Publishers (1980).

King's Fund Project Paper, *A Handbook for Nurse to Nurse Reporting*, London, King's Fund Centre (1979).

Kratz, C.R., *The Nursing Process*, London, Baillière Tindall (1979).

Long, R., *Systematic Nursing Care*, London, Faber & Faber (1981).

McFarlane, J.K., *Essays on Nursing*, London, King's Fund Centre, Project Paper RC2 (1980).

Nursing Times Booklet, *Rediscovering the patient* (supplement), vol. 74, no. 48 (1978).

Nursing Times Publication, *Teaching the Nursing Process*, London, Nursing Times (1977).

Nursing Times Publication, *Discharging Procedures*, London, Nursing Times (1980).

Roper N., Logan, W.W. and Tierney, A.J., *Learning to use the Process of Nursing*, Edinburgh, Churchill Livingstone (1981).

Royal College of Nursing, *Implementing the Nursing Process*, London, RCN (1979).

Royal College of Nursing, *Standards of Nursing Care*, London, RCN (1980).

Royal College of Nursing, *Towards Standards*, London, RCN (1981).

## Articles and comments

Alexander, M., 'Adapting the nursing process for use in a surgical unit', *Nursing Times,* vol. 75, no. 34, pp. 1443-1447 (1979).

Altschul, A.T., 'Use of the nursing process in psychiatric care', *Nursing Times,* vol. 73, no. 36, pp. 1412-1413 (1977).

Andrews, G.A., 'Complete nursing care – 2. The feelings of the ward sister', *Nursing Times,* vol. 76, no. 34, pp. 1484-1485 (1980).

Ashworth, P., 'Nursing process: a way to better care', *Nursing Mirror*, vol. 151, no. 9, pp. 26-27 (1980).

Ashworth, P., 'Nursing process – problems and solutions', *Nursing Mirror*, vol. 151, no. 10, pp. 34-36 (1980).

Ashworth, P. and Castledine, G., 'The way we teach nursing using the nursing process', *Medical Teacher*, vol. 3, no. 3, pp. 87-91 (1981).

Baines, L., 'Fully involved – an account of how a geriatric hospital is putting process into action', *Nursing Times*, vol. 77, no. 29, pp. 1262-1264 (1981).

Baldwin, S.M., 'Made to measure care', *Nursing Times*, vol. 72, no. 12, pp. 468-469 (1976).

Bendle, M., 'Confessions of a nursing process addict', *Community Outlook*, December, pp. 365-368 (1980).

Bond, C.A., 'A patient with Stevens-Johnson syndrome' (nursing process care study), *Nursing Times*, vol. 76, no. 46, pp. 2013-2015 (1980).

Brandrick, J., 'Nursing care study: a nursing care plan for convalescence following a cardiovascular accident', *Nursing Times*, vol. 76, no. 29, pp. 1253-1257 (1980).

Breckman, B., 'Who asks the processed patient?', *Nursing Mirror*, vol. 149, no. 15, p. 12 (1979).

Carter, S.L., 'Teaching the nursing process: the nurse educator', *Nursing Times*, vol. 75, no. 31, pp. 1315-1317 (1979).

Castledine, G., 'Nursing assessment of the musculoskeletal system', *Nursing*, June, 1st series, pp. 112-114 (1979).

Castledine, G., 'My nurse and my patient', *Nursing Mirror*, vol. 151, no. 6, p. 14 (1980).

Castledine, G., 'Forget the medical diagnosis', *Nursing Mirror*, vol. 151, no. 14, p. 12 (1980).

Castledine, G., 'Planning the patient's progress', *Nursing Mirror*, vol. 150, no. 13, p. 12 (1980).

Castledine, G., 'From one fellow to another, take better care', *Nursing Mirror*, vol. 151, no. 22, p. 12 (1980).

Castledine, G., 'The progress of "The Process"', *Nursing Mirror*, vol. 152, no. 6, p. 14 (1981).

Clark, M., 'Planning nursing care', *Nursing Times Occasional Paper*, vol. 74, no. 5, pp. 17-20 (1978).

Clark, M.O., 'The nursing process for practical reasons', *Nursing Times*, vol. 74, no. 48, pp. 1986-1987 (1978).

Collingwood, M.P., 'The nursing care plan', *Nursing Times Occasional Paper*, vol. 71, no. 12, pp. 21-22 (1975).

Cormack, D.F.S., 'The nursing process: an application of the SOPE model', *Nursing Times Occasional Paper*, vol. 76, no. 9, pp. 37-40 (1980).

Cowper-Smith, F., 'What is the point of the nursing process?' *Nursing Times*, vol. 74, no. 18, pp. 738-739 (1978).

Crow, J., 'The nursing process: theoretical background', *Nursing Times*, vol. 73, no. 24, pp. 892-896 (1977).

Crow, J., 'How and why to take a nursing history', *Nursing Times*, vol. 73, no. 25, pp. 950-957 (1977).

Crow. J., 'A nursing history questionnaire for two patients', *Nursing Times,* vol. 73, no. 26, pp. 978-982 (1977).

Darey, P.T., 'The nursing process – a base for all nursing developments', *Nursing Times,* vol. 76, no. 12, pp. 497-501 (1980). (This was a prize-winning essay.)

Davis, B.D., 'The nursing process for professional reasons', *Nursing Times,* vol. 74, no. 48, pp 1987-1988 (1978).

Duberley, J., 'How will the change strike me and you?', *Nursing Times,* vol. 73, no. 44, pp. 1736-1738 (1977).

Faulkner, A., 'Aye, there's the rub (communication skills and nursing process)', *Nursing Times,* vol. 77, no. 28, pp. 332-336 (1981).

Gooch, J.K., 'An experience of the nursing process', *Nursing Times,* vol. 77, no. 6, pp. 237-238 (1981).

Gooch, J.K., 'Change for the better', *Nursing Times,* vol. 77, no. 7, p. 264 (1981).

Grant, N., 'The nursing care plan 2', *Nursing Times Occasional Paper,* vol. 71, no. 12, pp. 21-22 (1975).

Grant, N., 'Time to care', London, Royal College of Nursing (1979).

Grubb, M., 'A clinical teacher's view of nursing process', *Nursing Times,* vol. 75, no. 34, pp. 1448-1449 (1979).

Hargreaves, I., 'The nursing process – the key to individualised care', *Nursing Times Occasional Paper,* vol. 71, no. 35, pp. 89-91 (1975).

Heath, J. 'It's a taxing process', *Nursing Mirror,* vol. 149, no. 8, pp. 24-27 (1979).

Hollingworth, S., 'A challenge for nurse teachers', *Nursing Times,* vol. 75, no. 30, p. 1263 (1979).

Holt, D. and Middleton, R., 'Making a new record', *Nursing Mirror,* vol. 151, no. 8, pp. 32-33 (1980).

Hunt, A., 'The individual approach' (nursing process in the operating dept), *Nursing Mirror,* vol. 149, no. 15, supplement (1979).

Jones, C., 'The nursing process – individualised care', *Nursing Mirror,* vol. 145, no. 15, pp. 13-14 (1977).

Jones, M.P., 'The nursing process in psychiatry', *Nursing Times,* vol. 76, no. 29, p. 1273 (1980).

Kershaw, K.E.M., 'Teaching the nursing process: standard care plan', *Nursing Times,* vol. 75, no. 33, pp. 1413-1416 (1979).

Kirwin, B., 'From the ivory tower to the ward floor', *Nursing Mirror,* vol. 150, no. 9, pp. 36-38 (1980).

Kratz, C., 'The nursing process', *Nursing Times,* vol. 73, no. 23, pp. 854-855 (1977).

Lowe, K.R., 'Hospital care of the elderly', *Nursing,* May, 1st series, pp. 1099-1101 (1981).

Luker, K.A. 'Teaching the nursing process'; 'A framework for the nursing process'; 'Problem orientated recordings', *Nursing Times,* vol. 75, no. 35, pp. 1488-1490 (1979).

McFarlane, J.K., 'A charter for caring', *Journal of Advanced Nursing,* vol. 1, no. 3, pp. 187-196 (1976).

McGilloway, F.A., 'The nursing process: a problem solving approach to patient care', *Int. Journal of Nursing Studies*, vol. 17, no. 2, pp. 29-90 (1980).

Mackie, L., 'Teaching the nursing process: revitalising the nursing care plan', *Nursing Times*, vol. 75, no. 34, pp. 1440-1442 (1979).

MacMillan, P., 'Please don't throw out the baby with the baby water', *Nursing Times*, vol. 75, no. 45, pp. 1923-1924 (1979).

Marks-Maran, D.J., 'Patient allocation *versus* task allocation', *Nursing Times*, vol. 74, no. 9, pp. 413-416 (1978).

Marks-Maran, D.J., 'In the process of better care', *Nursing Mirror*, vol. 149, no. 2, p. 12 (1979).

Marshall, S. 'A processed approach to Annie', *Nursing Mirror*, vol. 151, no. 11, supplement (1980).

Measures, A., 'The nursing process – a useful step', *Nursing Mirror*, vol. 148, no. 24, pp. 20-21 (1979).

Miller, A.E., 'Nurses' attitudes towards their patients', *Nursing Times*, vol. 75, no. 45, pp. 1929-1933 (1979).

Morland, R., 'Complete nursing care – 1', *Nursing Times*, vol. 76, no. 33, pp. 1426-1484 (1980).

Myers, N., 'Nursing diagnoses', *Nursing Times*, vol. 69, no. 38, pp. 1229-1230 (1973).

Neilson, A.F., Clarke, M.O. and Davis, B.D., 'Why do we need the nursing process?: for legal reasons, for practical reasons, for professional reasons', *Nursing Times*, vol. 74, no. 48, pp. 1984-1987 (1978).

Newall, E., 'The nursing process and nursing care studies', *Nursing Times*, vol. 76, no. 28, pp. 1235-1236 (1980).

Norton C., 'Assessing incontinence', *Nursing*, October, 1st series, pp. 789-791 (1980).

Nursing Times, 'A new concept of nursing: developed by a working group in Scotland', *Nursing Times*, vol. 72, no. 14, pp. 49-64 (1976).

O'Hare, E., 'The gingerbread man', *Nursing Times*, vol. 76, no. 8, pp. 318-320 (1980).

Pemberton, L., 'Nursing an unconscious patient', *Nursing Mirror*, vol. 149, no. 11, pp. 41-43 (1979).

Schurr, M., 'Getting it together', *Nursing Times*, vol. 75, no. 35, pp. 1472-1473 (1979).

Smith, L., 'A nursing history and data sheet (psychiatry)', *Nursing Times*, vol. 76, no. 13, pp. 749-754 (1980).

Sofaer, B., 'Spreading the word', *Nursing Times*, vol. 76, no. 13, pp. 567-568 (1980).

Syson-Nibbs, L., 'Progress through a planned approach', *Nursing Mirror*, vol. 150, no. 7, pp. 42-44 (1980).

Taylor, J., 'Introducing team nursing', *Nursing Times*, vol. 75, no. 47, pp. 2034-2037 (1979).

Thompson, A., 'Its value for special hospital patients', *Nursing Mirror*, vol. 148, no. 9, pp. 20-25 (1979).

Thompson, A., 'Applying the nursing process to the care of the mentally handicapped', *Nursing Mirror,* vol. 148, no. 10, pp. 26-28 (1979).

Thompson, J.N., 'The nursing process – handle with care', *Nursing Times,* vol. 75, no. 30, pp. 1261-1262 (1979).

Tucker, E.R., 'The nursing process', *Nursing Mirror,* vol. 149, no. 10, pp. 23-23 (1978).

Young, E.J., 'The teaching process', *Nursing Times,* vol. 76, no. 14, pp. 605-606 (1980).

## Nursing Times Series : The Nursing Process in Action

Baines, L., 'Fully involved (an account of how a geriatric hospital is putting process into action)', *Nursing Times,* vol. 77, no. 29, pp. 1262-1264 (1981).

Dale, J., 'A student's viewpoint', *Nursing Times,* vol. 77, no. 26, p. 1131 (1981).

Keane, P., 'The nursing process in a psychiatric context', *Nursing Times,* vol. 77, no. 28, pp. 1223-1224 (1981).

Kershaw, K.E.M., 'Teaching and evaluating care', *Nursing Times,* vol. 77, no. 26, pp. 1126-1128 (1981).

Leslie, F. and Shiells, E., 'The nursing process related to mental handicap care', *Nursing Times,* vol. 77, no. 27, pp. 1169-1174 (1981).

Lewis, M., 'The teaching programme', *Nursing Times,* vol. 77, no. 26, pp. 1128-1131 (1981).

Norton, D., 'The quiet revolution: introduction of the nursing process in a region', *Nursing Times,* vol. 77, no. 25, pp. 1067-1069 (1981).

Robertson, R., 'The nursing process in community nursing', *Nursing Times,* vol. 77, no. 30, pp 1299-1304 (1981).

# References

Ashworth, P.M. and Castledine, G. (1980). *Joint Service/Education Appointments in Nursing,* Issues in Nurse Education, *Medical Teacher,* vol. 2, no. 6.

Ashworth, P.M., Castledine, G. and McFarlane, J.K. (1978). *The Process in Practice,* Nursing Times Supplement — Rediscovering the Patient, London, Macmillan.

Bates, B. (1979). *A Guide to Physical Examination,* 2nd edn, Philadelphia, J.B. Lippincott.

Becknell, E.P. and Smith D.M. (1975). *System of Nursing Practice,* Philadelphia, F.A. Davis.

Black, D. (Chairman) (1980). *Report of the Working Group on Inequalities in Health,* Department of Health and Social Security, London, HMSO.

Blicharz, M. (1979). 'Interventions that promote decubiti healing', in Kennedy, M.S. and Pfeifer, G.M., Eds., *Current Practice in Nursing Care of the Adult,* St Louis, C.V. Mosby.

Bower, F.L. (1972). *The Process of Planning Nursing Care,* St Louis, C.V. Mosby.

Castledine, G. *et al.* (1981). 'The nursing process and standards of care', *JAN Forum, Journal of Advanced Nursing,* vol. 6, pp. 503–514.

Ciske, K.L. (1974). 'Primary nursing: an organisation that promotes professional practice' (Reprinted 1977 in a reader on Primary Nursing, by the *Journal of Nursing Administration,* and published by Contemporary Pub. Inc., Wakefield, Massachusetts).

Ciske, K.L. (1979). 'Accountability — the essence of primary nursing', *American Journal of Nursing,* vol. 79, no. 5, p. 890.

Davies, C. (Ed.) (1980). *Rewriting Nursing History,* London, Croom Helm.

Department of Health and Social Security (1972). *Report of the Committee on Nursing,* Prof. Asa Briggs (Chairman), National Health Service, Cmnd. 5115, London, HMSO.

Dunn, H.L. (1958). 'Positive wellness in the human natural posture', Development Note no. 58, DAP-7, p. 3, Washington D.C. (government document; also in *American Journal of Public Health,* vol. 49, p. 788, June 1959).

Dunn, H.L. (1961). *High-level Wellness,* p. 4. Arlington, Beatty.

Durand, M. and Prince R. (1966). 'Nursing diagnosis; process and decision', *Nursing Forum,* vol. V, pp. 50-64.

Edinburg, G.M., Zinberg, N.E. and Kelman, W. (1975). *Clinical Interviewing and Counselling: Principles and Techniques,* New York, Appleton Century Croft.

Ganong, J. and Ganong, W. (1977). 'Evaluating staff performance', in *Current Perspectives in Nursing Management* (Ed. Ann Marriner), St Louis, C.V. Mosby.

Guy's Hospital (1981). 'Organic mental impairment in the elderly', *Journal of Royal College of Physicians of London,* vol. 15, no. 3.

Henderson, V. (1966). *The Nature of Nursing*, London, Collier Macmillan.

Kratz, C. (1979). 'Primary nursing — letter from Australia', *Nursing Times*, vol. 75, no. 42, pp. 1790–1791.

Lalonde, M. (1974). *A New Perspective on the Health of Canadians*, Ottawa, Government of Canada.

Larkin, P.D. and Backer, B.A. (1977). *Problem Oriented Nursing Assignment*, New York, McGraw-Hill.

Lee, M. (1979). 'Towards better care: primary nursing', *Nursing Times Occasional Paper*, vol. 75, no. 51.

Lelean, S.R. (1973). 'Ready for report nurse?', *Study of Nursing Care Project Reports*, series 2, no. 2, London, RCN.

McCain, F.R. (1965). 'Nursing by assessment — not intuition', *American Journal of Nursing*, vol. 65, no. 4, pp. 82–83.

McCarthy, M.M. (1981). 'The nursing process: application of current thinking in clinical problem solving', *Journal of Advanced Nursing*, vol. 6, pp. 173–177.

MacKenzie Davey, D. and McDonnell, P. (1975). *How to Interview*, British Institute of Management, Halifax and London, Edward Mortimer Ltd.

Manthey, M., Ciske, K., Robertson, P. and Harris, I. (1970). 'Primary nursing — a return to the concept of "my nurse and my patient" ', *Nursing Forum*, vol. 9(1), pp. 65–83.

Marram, G.D. (1979). 'Primary nursing', in *Current Perspectives in Nursing Management* (Ed. Ann Marriner), St Louis, C.V. Mosby.

Maslow, A.H. (1943). 'A theory of human motivation', *Psychological Review*, vol. 5, pp. 370–396.

Maslow, A.H. (1954). *Motivation and Personality*, New York, Harper and Row.

Mayers, M.G. (1978). *A Systematic Approach to the Nursing Care Plan*, 2nd edn, New York, Appleton Century Croft.

Norton, D. (1975). *An Investigation of Geriatric Nursing Problems in Hospital*, Edinburgh, Churchill Livingstone.

Orem, D. (1980). *Nursing: Concepts of Practice*, 2nd edn, New York, McGraw-Hill.

President's Commission on the Health Needs of the Nation (1953). *Building America's Health*, vol. 2, Washington D.C., US Government Printing Office.

Weed, L.L. (1970). *Medical Records, Medical Education and Patient Care*, Chicago, Year Book.

Wolff, H. and Erickson, R. (1977). 'The Assessment Man'. *Nursing Outlook*, vol. 25, no. 2.

World Health Organisation (1947). 'Constitution of the W.H.O.', *Chronicle of the World Health Organisation*, vol. 1, pp.1–2 (Geneva).

# Index

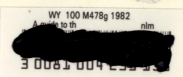